DEFY AGING
Make the Rest of Your Life
the Best of Your Life

JACOB ROSENSTEIN, M.D.

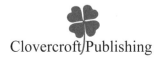
Clovercroft Publishing

Defy Aging

Published by Clovercroft Publishing, Franklin, Tennessee in association with OnFire Marketing

Edited by Tammy Kling and Tiarra Tompkins

Cover design by Brightly

Interior Design by Adept Content Solutions

ISBN: Hardcover 978-1-945507-88-5
          Paperback 978-1-945507-89-2

Printed in the United States of America

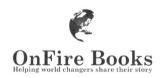

OnFire Books
Helping world changers share their story

In the end, it's not the years in your life that count—it's the life in your years.

Anonymous

CONTENTS

Diseases can rarely be eliminated through early diagnosis or good treatment, but prevention can eliminate disease.

Denis Burkitt

FOREWORD

Six years ago, I felt my energy level take a dramatic dive.

Although I was only thirty, years of endless insomnia, brutally long work hours, and late-night carousing had finally caught up with me, breaking my resolve and threatening to knock my productivity down to a sluggish pace.

As a recent law school grad from an overachieving family, I had embarked on a mission to find professional nirvana, building my own real estate investment company and launching two start-ups with a tenacity that bordered on insane. I worked, imbibed, and then paced frenetically during sleepless nights as though high-octane fuel coursed through my veins, propelling me to chase some elusive state of everlasting fulfillment. But the reality was I was running on fumes.

I was driven by some misguided notion that I needed to be someone better, my choices probably dictated more by angry determination to prove something to the world, my family, or myself than any true desire to self-improve. My life was like an ongoing Olympic event to fill something that no one could see and probably didn't exist. That took a toll on my health in ways I couldn't imagine.

Like a toxic well threatening to overflow, I was no longer able to suppress the ailments accumulating inside me. I battled migraines and was wracked by bouts of anxiety and depression. I had always been trim, but my body composition began to deteriorate. My weight fluctuated in a back-and-forth, gain-and-loss cycle. I developed dark circles under my eyes, my skin became cracked and dehydrated, and my thick black hair had begun to thin. My insides were in chaos, like a war zone.

By the time I made it to my doctor, my cholesterol was obscenely high, my testosterone was unusually low, and my estrogen depleted. I had a number of vitamin deficiencies. In the past, I had sought medical treatment to surgically remove gynecomastia, enlarged breast tissue that I had tried to hide for years with distorted posture, a habit that became a chronic source of pain.

My lifestyle was buoyed by prescriptions for stimulants and sedatives that medically manipulated my sleep patterns and artificially controlled my attention span. I was irritable, and my marriage began to feel the strain. With no antidote in sight, I plunged deeper into destructive cycles, immersing myself further in work with an intensity that obscured my view of a better life ahead.

Then, five years ago, my daughter was born. I remember peering into her tiny face, seeing her eyes struggling to take in the world, and becoming numb with fear. I sobbed, wondering how I would care for her if I couldn't take care of myself. Then, the despair loosened its grip and a calmness came over me. I felt myself become anchored and reclaimed a purpose in life. In an instant, my outlook changed, and I started to ask myself new questions.

I became hell-bent on discovering the root of my health problems, applying the same hyper-discipline and fierce tenacity to investigating my mental and physical well-being that I had for my business ventures. I read every health book I could find. I gave up meat and was tested for allergies. I visited hyperbaric chambers. I tried cryotherapy, transcendental meditation, and sensory deprivation. I even had vitamin C injected intravenously three times a week. But despite my best efforts and thorough assessment, nothing seemed to alleviate my symptoms.

Then, about a year ago, a friend introduced me to Dr. Jacob Rosenstein as a potential business partner. An anti-aging expert and talented neurosurgeon with a brilliant business mind, he struck me with his ability to attain great success by helping others. We became fast friends. It didn't take long for him to inquire about my health. He asked questions, and they were detailed, probing questions that no one had asked before.

He wanted to know about my baseline and how I knew whether a certain treatment was working. I explained that I had relied on the simple gauge of my gut feeling. He responded that our feelings can lie. He then peppered me with nuanced questions, carefully evaluating each answer. He observed that I had approached my health assessment like a blind person throwing darts at the wall, trying everything imaginable without establishing a way to measure the results and in some cases completely misfiring. The gynecomastia, I learned, was caused by hormonal problems that could have been treated medically instead of through surgery. I realized I had been doing it all wrong.

That began my journey through Dr. Rosenstein's program, which teaches people how to reduce stress, prevent disease, and live longer through the simple process of adopting healthy lifestyle choices, such as exercising and adhering to a nutritional diet.

But his program does not merely examine the surface; it begins with an executive health evaluation that analyzes medical history, mental clarity, sexual health, risk factors, fitness, lifestyle, and hormone levels. In a methodical, forensic-like assessment that works from the inside out, Dr. Rosenstein conducts extensive blood work to measure data in ninety different biomarkers, and he captures a three-dimensional image of your carotid artery to assess the thickness of the arterial wall and plaque formation. He tests your fitness level, grip strength, flexibility, and balance, as well as your brain function and cognitive ability. With those and a slew of other tests, he develops a treatment plan, based on your specific needs. Then, he uses the test results to customize pharmaceutical-grade supplements, determining exact hormonal, vitamin, and mineral levels needed for each patient. The treatment plan and supplement levels are then adjusted through periodic blood screens.

I eagerly submitted to the battery of tests, handing over twelve vials of my blood for the most comprehensive medical exam I'd ever had. Dr. Rosenstein checked the density of every bone in my body. He looked for signs of body misalignment, osteoporosis, and spinal degeneration. He discovered that I was prediabetic and detected a number of moderate food allergies causing inflammation, including eggs, dairy, turmeric, and tilapia. I began a high-nutrition diet of lean protein, fruits, and vegetables, and I eliminated high-sugar, allergy-inducing, and processed foods. I incorporated his exercise regime and began taking daily supplements that had been customized for me.

The transformation was incredible. My energy level went through the roof. My skin cleared up and returned to its healthy, even glow, and my hair regained its thickness. My body composition came down to a healthy level. I disposed of my prescription drugs and began sleeping eight hours a night. My marriage improved, and my business started booming. My wife and I are now in the program together, and planning family meals has become a central focus of our marriage. My mind found a pathway to my body, and my days as a feral saboteur were over.

Now, as a radiating convert embracing a new way of life, I recall something powerful Dr. Rosenstein said to me. He said, "Ari, your body is like an orchestra. You have flutes, cellos, violins, drums, and accordions, all playing their different parts. And I am the greatest conductor in the world."

I know how one violin string left untuned can mar an entire orchestra, just as one biochemical imbalance can set our bodies completely off course. It doesn't matter what your goal is—the truth is, you will never reach it if you're not healthy. With our own modulated orchestra where our biological, physiological, and psychological systems strike a perfect harmony, we can master each crescendo, syncopated beat, or trill that comes our way. For me, Dr. Rosenstein accomplished the unthinkable. He cracked the code to my health and helped me restore my vitality, as if to irrigate and fine-tune each one of my cells for peak performance. He is, indeed, a maestro of his own making, one who helped me make my music play again. And for anyone else who wants to make life's music again, this is one opus you won't want to miss.

Ari Rastegar
CEO, Rastegar Equity Partners

Everyone is so unique and different that I have never seen two cases be exactly alike in over 11,000 surgeries. We are all so different yet so much alike.

Dr. Jacob Rosenstein

INTRODUCTION

Good health doesn't happen by accident.

In fact, nothing in life does. It takes work to maintain our cars, our houses, and our careers, and many people do. When I see someone in my office as a patient, after spending some time with them taking an extensive history, it often becomes apparent that I have my work cut out for me. Typically, they've taken such poor care of their bodies that it's a challenge to reverse the process. They've paid attention to everything in life except their health.

They've taken care of their family, their business, their spouse, their kids, their employees, their friends, and their neighbors, but often they have completely ignored their own health. Many people simply don't know what good health looks and feels like. They have forgotten, too entrenched in life's daily chores, too busy to pay attention, and taking too little time. By the time a patient enters my office, it has been years of cumulative bad lifestyle choices, poor eating habits, a sedentary lifestyle, not enough exercise, and maybe a little too much alcohol or tobacco. All these contribute and have a direct impact on modern-day maladies and diseases.

This is especially true for cardiovascular diseases (heart attacks and strokes). This single category is responsible for more deaths and disability in both men and women than any other. In the United States in 2014, more people died of cardiovascular disease than cancer, which also is a lifestyle disease (747,451 v. 591,699).

GETTING THERE STARTS WITH AWARENESS THAT YOU MAY NOT BE FUNCTIONING AS WELL AS YOU SHOULD BE, NEED TO BE, OR WANT TO BE.

Diabetes was responsible for another 76,488. Thus 1,415,638 deaths, or 54 percent of all deaths, were related directly to heart disease, stroke, and diabetes. The formula for poor health is simple. Bad food choices combined with a sedentary lifestyle equals a negative outcome. It is not just a possibility but a certainty. Continue with poor lifestyle habits and unhealthy living, and your fate is sealed.

The road you are heading down is not a pretty one. I've seen it, lived it, treated it, and experienced it.

So why don't people change? For some they simply don't know any better. They follow the example set by their family and friends. For others, they may have an idea that their lifestyle habits may not be the best, but it is too difficult to change.

Change takes effort. Effort takes energy. Energy is usually lacking, so not much happens. It is a downward spiral. The worse your diet, the more sedentary you become. The more sedentary you become, the less energy you have. The less energy you have, the less likely you are to change for the better. Energy, boundless energy, is the key to success in life.

The onset and progression of poor health is insidious in nature. Poor health doesn't happen overnight. You don't even notice your declining health in the beginning. It festers day in and day out with every poor food choice and continues year after year for decades. Often, even with progression, people don't see the decline because the changes occur so slowly and subtly. But gradually they start to lose their health, vigor, and vitality.

By that point, they've accepted a new normal and have adapted to it. Maybe they're out of breath with achy muscles and joints or cannot climb stairs. They begin to move slower, all the while attributing it to normal aging.

People often forget what it feels like to feel healthy and strong, full of life, full of passion, and full of boundless energy. They forget what it is to be engaged and interacting with the world! Having forgotten what the real normal is like, they begin to accept a lower level of function, and it continues to get worse and worse over time. People are left feeling exhausted at the end of the day, coming home and crashing on the couch with a remote control and falling asleep. But it doesn't have to be this way.

I've spent years studying how and why we age, and after decades seeing patients, I decided to help educate the general public. Year after year, I saw unhealthy people walk into my office who put their business priorities ahead of their own health. Year after year, I witnessed otherwise smart people remain uninformed and uneducated about their bodies. This book is a compilation of the things I've learned over many years of study and practice about health, wellness, aging, and disease in order to help you focus on getting your health and mojo back. An ounce of prevention is worth a pound of cure. So, the sooner you incorporate living a healthier lifestyle and start making healthier food choices, the sooner you will see the results.

What if we could turn back time? It turns out it is possible to biologically rewind the clock of accelerated aging, but to do so, you must first understand what is happening when you age and why. There are certain things that are happening as we age that are reversible, and that is what we will concentrate on. Why age any faster than you have to?

The truth is, you don't have to age like your unhealthy predecessors. If you make smarter and healthier lifestyle choices and manage, correct, and reverse what is reversible as you grow older, you can live well into your nineties and beyond. Many of today's diseases that lead to death, disability, frailty, and feebleness are preventable.

Unfortunately, most people do not realize this and accept a progressive declining level of function as they get older, attributing it to "normal aging." Normal aging should not be synonymous with frailty, feebleness, and loss of function. Just because you are getting older does not mean you cannot live life to the fullest with vigor, vitality, and boundless energy. I am currently in my sixties and feel better, look better, function better, and have better surgical skills than when I was in my twenties and thirties.

The aches and pains that developed in my forties are totally gone. Image—no aches or pains. How many in their sixties can say that? I wake up every morning feeling refreshed, full of energy, and ready to take on the day. I'll put in a full day's work, often performing complicated surgeries that can last ten hours, yet I still have the energy to exercise and work out after these long cases. That is the meaning of boundless energy: the ability to do whatever you want, whenever you want, and not feel tired and exhausted at the end of the day.

SINCE INFLAMMATION IS ONE OF THE FOUNDATIONAL CAUSES OF DISEASE AND PAIN IN THE BODY, CONTROLLING IT IS EXTREMELY IMPORTANT.

I have been a high energy guy ever since I can remember. When I was a young child, people would say to me, "You have so much energy." I never knew what they were talking about until I lost it. It was then that I realized what they meant. I had turned fifty, and suddenly, I found myself falling asleep while writing post-op orders in the recovery room. Exercising afterward was out of the question. I was getting home and crashing on the couch. My energy was gone, and I was not happy about it. It final-ly dawned on me what was happening: I was getting old. As I was not ready yet to put down the scalpel, I started to research what happens to our bodies as we age. That is when I discovered that it is not hopeless. There are a lot of things that can be done to slow down and even reverse the aging process.

Why We Age

As you get older, there are certain things that occur in your body that you can do something about—and others that you can't. We need to focus on those things we can change and influence.

A simple piece of advice I once heard: "If you want to stay healthy, stay away from sick people!" So, if you want to avoid an infection such as the flu, meningitis, or pneumonia, stay away from infected people.

While true for infectious diseases, especially if you are immune compromised, this is really not practical when you are a doctor or healthcare worker. The Ebola epidemic showed us just how quickly things can get out of control. In the same vein, if every-one around you is practicing and exhibiting poor lifestyle choices (drugs, alcohol, tobacco, poor diet, sedentary lifestyle), it may be hard to break away and do what is needed to regain your health and to slow down or even reverse the aging process.

So, what is it that makes us age? I did not say grow old, but I said *age!*

Inflammation—chronic inflammation, that is—is a big one! It slowly destroys our bodies from the inside out, affecting every or-gan and tissue in our body. The good news is that inflammation is controllable and reversible. You might be wondering just how exactly we do that. Diet and exercise (especially diet) are key to reversing this process.

The truth is that most people are not aware that the aches and pains they feel as they get older are directly related to chronic inflammation. Not knowing the root causes and thinking it is normal aging, they learn to adjust to it the best they can, rather than trying to reverse the process. In the meantime, ongoing damage to their bodies is occurring. Food can be medicine, or food can be poison. You determine which it is by what you put in your mouth. If you eat the wrong foods, it will make you old and sick fast.

Our Main Weapon against Inflammation Is Our Diet

Eating the right foods can fight inflammation and eliminate the gradual decay of our bodies caused by free radicals. Free radicals are unstable molecules produced as normal byproducts of energy production and metabolism in our cells. In a healthy situation, free radicals are neutralized by antioxidants before they can do damage to our bodies. Our bodies produce some antioxidants; the rest we must get through our diet. Free radicals attack our cells, cell membranes, cellular organelles, and DNA, causing damage and accelerated aging. Bad foods exacerbate the process, while good foods are preventive. There is a constant battle between free radical production and free radical neutralization.

When there is an imbalance between free radical production and the ability of the body to detoxify them through antioxidants, an unhealthy situation is created known as oxidative stress. Oxidative stress is a major factor associated with chronic disease and aging. The less excess free radicals you have, the healthier you are. The less oxidative stress, the healthier you will be and the longer you will live.

We can help our bodies fight free radicals by making the right food choices consistently over time and rejecting things like sugar, processed foods, simple carbohydrates, and sweets. You never know what hidden toxins might be present in processed foods.

More on that later, but the primary reason for calling attention to this fact right now is that most people know they need to eat healthy or perhaps they've been taught that at some point in their lives, yet the incidence of diabetes and obesity continues to climb and remains at an all-time high. Why is this? Is it lack of knowledge, lack of time, being too busy to educate yourself or too comfortable and set in your ways, finding it too hard to change, or is it unintentional? You think you are eating healthy, but you are not. Often it takes a crisis for someone to finally realize it's time to change their life. How about you? No matter where you are on the health span spectrum, this book can help. Whether you're fit and want to get fitter, young or middle-aged and want to turn back the hands of time, or facing a health crisis, the information inside this book can be a wakeup call. It's your choice.

Today is the first day of the rest of your life. Will you make the commitment to make positive changes and form life-changing habits?

Someone asked me during the writing of this book, "What are the top five worst foods for your body?" You may be surprised by the answer. Ask the average person and their reply will be diet sweeteners, chocolate, or sugar. Those are the obvious offenders, which is why most people aren't even aware when they're eating and sabotaging their health and their fitness regimen.

My answer was:

Bread
Bread
Bread
Bread
and
Bread

You should have seen the look on their face! Most people are surprised to learn that even whole wheat bread is unhealthy for you. Bread metabolizes into sugar, and *sugar* is your enemy. Sugar makes you old. Sugar makes you fat. And sugar is hidden in everything.

But sugar doesn't only come from sweets, candy, and chocolate. It comes from many foods you never would have thought would contain sugar. Eating a potato can spike your blood sugar. Eating bread will spike your blood sugar, and it will remain elevated for longer than you think. This will, in turn, cause fat to accumulate around your middle. The more you eat sugar, either obvious or hidden in a food, the bigger your stomach will grow. If you don't want fat around your belly and you want to be able to see those abs you've worked so hard for, you've got to eat differently and eliminate all sources of sugar, hidden or otherwise.

THE ONSET AND PROGRESSION OF POOR HEALTH IS INSIDIOUS IN NATURE.

POOR HEALTH DOESN'T HAPPEN OVERNIGHT.

When you eat a carb, always balance it with a protein or fat to decrease the spike in blood sugar that occurs as a result. It also makes a difference in the order you eat it. Sequence matters. Eat the protein and fat first. Eat your carbs last. I'll explain why as we get deeper into the book, but how we eat, what we eat, and when we eat it *matters*.

In the book you're about to read, you'll see why I empha-size aging from the inside out versus the outside in. This is a distinction from many anti-aging doctors who are focused on the exterior. I'm not an anti-aging doctor, and I'm not focused on the exterior. I'm a neurosurgeon who has looked inside people's bodies for decades, observing their arteries, fat, muscle, and the damage that clogged arteries cause. I'm an anti-aging advocate who focuses on health and wellness because I've seen what happens to unhealthy people and the damage they do to themselves. I changed my own life, and so can you. I'm here to show you what really works.

Year after year, I see patients and give them advice, but unfortunately sometimes they never take it. To be able to change, you must want to change. To do the same thing repeatedly and expect a different result is widely recognized as insanity. It's painful to see people ill and sick, especially when you know there are answers, preventive measures, and changes in lifestyle that could very literally cure them. It is very difficult to know you can change someone's life, increase their life span, and increase their quality of life, yet they are unwilling to do what it takes to turn their health around.

I encourage you to ask yourself these questions:

What do you want your health now and in the future to be?

What would you like your level of function now and in the future to be?

Throughout this book, I will teach you how to age well with vigor and vitality!

The greatest wealth is health.

Virgil

CHAPTER 1

DEFYING AGE: HOW TO LIVE TO ONE HUNDRED

On my first day of medical school at Johns Hopkins University, all of us students were gathered in a large auditorium eager to get started. The dean of the medical school, Dr. Richard Ross, came out to welcome us all to Hopkins. It was an exciting and energetic moment!

One thing he said has always stuck with me: "Half of what you are going to learn over the next four years is wrong. The problem is we don't know which half." What he was saying that day was to always keep an open mind and to continue to grow and learn and add to our knowledge base. It is only with time that we would be able to figure out which half of what we learned those four years was correct and which half was wrong. And I've discovered that the same thing is true with most things in life. As you travel on your own life path, you'll learn, grow, discover, and learn some more. The things you learned a decade ago may not work in your present-day experience. You may have to apply new knowledge. Technology or circumstances may have changed. Life is about being open to the possibility of learning new things.

Medicine is a fantastic profession because it never gets old. You are always and forever learning. As it turns out, a lot of what we thought we knew about aging was not quite what we thought at all. Each and every year, there have been new developments, new discoveries, and incredible findings based on the way people live and die. The most remarkable discovery of all for many people is that your aging can largely be determined by the choices you make. Many people travel through life on autopilot without understanding their bodies until they slow down or are stricken with illness. They attribute this all to the aging process. But it simply doesn't have to be that way. I've changed my life, and you can too!

I EMPHASIZE AGING FROM THE INSIDE OUT VERSUS THE OUTSIDE IN. THIS IS A DISTINCTION FROM MANY ANTI-AGING DOCTORS WHO ARE FOCUSED ON THE EXTERIOR. I'M NOT AN ANTI-AGING DOCTOR, AND I'M NOT FOCUSED ON THE EXTERIOR. I'M A NEUROSURGEON WHO HAS LOOKED INSIDE PEOPLE'S BODIES FOR DECADES, OBSERVING THEIR ARTERIES, FAT, MUSCLE, AND THE DAMAGE THAT CLOGGED ARTERIES CAUSE.

I've made it my life's work to understand the human body.

Not many people can say they get to see the inside of the human body on a nearly daily basis, but I do in surgery. As a neurosurgeon, I've operated on a variety of patients from all walks of life: from royalty to the homeless and in various states of health; from the nearly dead to the elite athlete; and of many body types, from the lean and trim to the morbidly obese. It's not hard to figure out who will be your ideal patient for surgery and who will be your worst nightmare. When it comes to surgery, size matters. The more overweight or obese you are, the more difficult it is for a surgeon to do his job.

You have to get to your target in order to do the operation you came to do. Quite simply, the further away from your skin surface that target is, the deeper it is and the harder it is to get to. In the thirty-seven years that I have been doing surgery, our surgical instruments have gotten longer and longer as the population has gotten bigger and bigger.

The bigger you get, the more fat you have accumulating around your organs. The more fat accumulating in your belly, the sicker you become because fat accumulation in your abdomen creates a very dangerous situation in terms of your long-term health. There's no hiding fat. There's no concealing years of damage that unhealthy eating and a sedentary lifestyle have created. Humans are their own worst enemies, more so than the environment.

Life Cycles

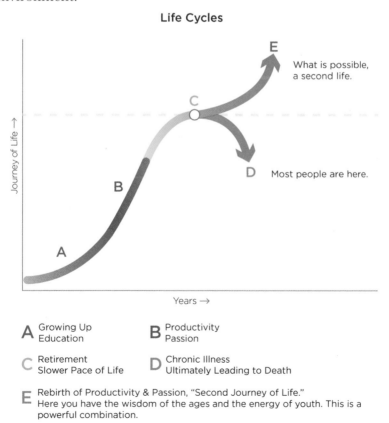

A Growing Up
   Education

B Productivity
   Passion

C Retirement
   Slower Pace of Life

D Chronic Illness
   Ultimately Leading to Death

E Rebirth of Productivity & Passion, "Second Journey of Life."
   Here you have the wisdom of the ages and the energy of youth. This is a
   powerful combination.

Each one of us has been given the freedom of choice, including the freedom to choose our own destiny and the freedom to make daily decisions about what we will eat, how much soda or sugar we will ingest, and how much inflammation or limited mobility we are willing to put up with. I hope this book is an eye opener and a wakeup call for anyone who has been living with chronic pain and disease caused by lack of exercise and a poor diet. Today is a new day. Let's work together to make immediate changes to transform and extend your life. You may not aspire to live to one hundred, but you can certainly live a better, longer, and more active life than ever before.

Seeing the dramatic results on a daily basis that my patients have achieved by putting in place simple lifestyle changes continues to be an inspiration for my own personal quest to defy aging. I want to show you how you can regain energy, increase muscle mass, reduce belly fat, and gain a new and more youthful appearance and outlook on life! It's not about how long you live but how well you live. It's not your chronologic age that matters but your biologic age. It's about aging well, aging strong, reducing inflammation, increasing your energy to higher levels than ever before, and reclaiming your youthful outlook on life. I'm not a plastic surgeon promoting anti-aging from the outside in. Anti-aging, in fact, occurs from the inside out.

Plastic surgeons may not like the facts that we talk about inside this book at all—because I educate people how to age well from the inside out. My approach is real, not a façade, not lipstick, and not "plastic."

The truth is that there are specific things you can do to take control of your health, and you can start today. I see patients every day who exhibit the ravages of poor lifestyle choices on their bodies. It affects every organ that we have: our heart, our brain, our liver, our blood vessels, our muscle, our bones, our skin, and our joints. You name the organ: it is affected through the accumulation of poor choices on the body.

Often, I'm asked, "How can one prevent aging, and turn back the hands of time?"

Prevention Is the Cure

It is not uncommon for me to see patients after they have experienced the consequences of poor lifestyle choices. They are sometimes distressed after receiving a negative diagnosis and want to understand how to get healthy again. Over the years, I have helped a lot of people regain their health and look and feel better. I have been successful in doing this as I know what I am doing having been there myself.

When you glance at my before-and-after pictures in the back of this book, you'll see that I walk the talk. Some patients have made so many poor choices over decades that the damage can be far more difficult to reverse, but it's never too late start. I mention this because the very best thing you can do for your health right now is to start an anti-aging lifestyle today. The sooner the better. Don't be the person damaging their body and promoting inflammation on a daily basis. Be the one who is promoting health from the inside out, striving for boundless energy and youthful skin by making healthy food choices, supplementing with nutritional supplements and vitamins to fill in any gaps present in your diet, and exercising vigorously on a regular basis.

NO MATTER HOW OLD YOU ARE, PREVENTION IS THE KEY AND THE CURE.

The less damage to your body, the longer it will last. Focus on preventing decline in all areas.

You may not want to live to one hundred, always fearing frailty and feebleness, but there's certainly a lot you can do to extend your health span, which is that period of time when you are in optimal health free of chronic disease and functioning at your best, both physically and mentally.

IT'S POSSIBLE TO SLOW DOWN AND EVEN REVERSE THE AGING PROCESS, UNDO SOME OF THE DAMAGE, AND REJUVENATE YOUR BODY, ORGANS, CELLS AND TELOMERES (MORE ON THAT LATER). AND YOU CAN START TODAY!

The simplest response I have when patients ask me what they can do to defy aging is to advise patients to (a) start exercising and eating right and (b) enter my age-management program for an in-depth evaluation where I cover every aspect of their health and lifestyle and formulate a personalized treatment plan, including appropriate nutritional supplements where needed.

I'll talk a lot about telomeres, our cellular time keepers; nutrition; exercise; and hormones as well as nutritional supplements in the pages to follow and why some nutraceuticals and vitamins are absolutely essential to turning back the hands of time.

The Brain, Vascular System, and Skin

Sometimes people come to see me and they're worried about declining cognitive function from diseases such as Alzheimer's or dementia. The answer to preventing dementia and brain-related diseases is the same answer I give for preventing physical ailments and diseases: Exercise regularly, avoid sugar, eat smart, supplement with vitamins and nutraceuticals, and focus on really reducing inflammation.

Nourish your brain and your whole body with whole, real, natural, and healthy foods as well as vitamins, minerals, trace elements, and selective nutritional supplements.

Exercised and educated brains work better and function longer than brains that remain idle. Blood flow, inflammation, and free radical damage are key reasons the brain "ages" (becomes sluggish and poorly responsive). I tell my patients to continually challenge their brain (and body). It's good for you!

Certain nutritional supplements, such as fish oil, can make a difference when it comes to brain health. Nutritional deficiencies can cause cognitive dysfunction. So, if you are experiencing memory loss, make sure you don't have a nutrient or vitamin deficiency. Nutritional supplements and vitamins help to fill the gaps that might be present in your diet. It's important to make up for it by taking the proper supplements and vitamins. You can begin living a healthier lifestyle with proper supplementation today.

WHILE I CAN SHOW YOU THE WAY, IT IS UP TO YOU TO MAKE IT HAPPEN. THIS IS NOT A SPECTATOR SPORT. YOUR ACTIVE PARTICIPATION IS ESSENTIAL IF YOU ARE TO GET THE RESULTS THAT YOU ARE LOOKING FOR.

Nutrition and exercise are the answers for fighting off dementia and Alzheimer's and preventing any additional damage. Don't forget that the brain is just like any other organ. Without the proper nutrients and oxygen, it becomes inflamed, damaged, and old. In our age-management practice, we provide very specific and individualized programs with personalized nutritional supplements, including my very special and proprietary *Vitamere Ultra Anti Aging Multivitamin* which contains not only the essential vitamins, minerals, and trace elements of a multipurpose multivitamin, but also ingredients that promote DNA health and telomere length, which are important in reversing cellular aging.

Is It Possible to Live to One Hundred?

Now more than ever, extending lifespan and living well beyond the ninth decade is possible. It's an exciting time to be alive! Studies of centenarians and even super-centenarians are revealing. They show us how this unique population lives to defy aging.

In an article in *Neuroscience News* titled "How to Live to 100: Scientists Crack the Secrets of Centenarians," they reported that centenarians and their offspring had less inflammation than the general population.

The good news is that most people who suffer from inflammation can reverse it with proper diet and nutrition, and it can be reversed quickly. Inflammation is a key indicator of health and disease, and it's something we have control over if we make the right choices. Many people live in a constant inflamed state, not knowing that they have the power and ability to reverse this.

> THE BRAIN IS AN ORGAN. NO AMOUNT OF CROSSWORD PUZZLES CAN PREVENT AGING IN AN ALREADY-DAMAGED OR UNHEALTHY BODY PART. YOU'VE GOT TO FEED YOUR BODY AND FEED YOUR BRAIN.

Professor Thomas von Zglinicki, from Newcastle University's Institute for Ageing, led the UK part of the study. He said, "Centenarians and supercentenarians are different—put simply, they age slower. They can ward off diseases for much longer than the general population."

In groups of people aged 105 and over (semi-supercentenarians), those 100 to 104 (centenarians), and those nearly 100 and their offspring, the team measured a number of health markers which they believe contribute toward successful aging, including blood cell numbers, metabolism, liver and kidney function, inflammation, and telomere length.

The article noted that scientists expected to see a continuous shortening of telomeres with age, but what they found was that the children of centenarians, who have a good chance of becoming centenarians themselves, maintained their telomeres at a "youthful" level corresponding to about sixty years of age even when they became eighty or older.

What's a Telomere?

Chances are you've already read articles about telomeres, but the short definition is that telomeres are structures found at the ends of our chromosomes. They keep the strands of DNA from unraveling. You can think of them as the plastic tips at the ends of your shoelaces that keep the shoelaces from unraveling. They consist of the same short DNA sequence, repeated over and over again. When you are born, your telomere length is at its longest. Each time a cell divides, the telomere length gets shorter and shorter. Eventually the telomere length gets so short that the cell can no longer divide, and the cell reaches senescence or dies. The longer your telomeres are, the younger your cells are, and the younger you are in terms of biologic age. Telomere length has been used as a marker of biologic age. There are several scientific studies and articles that indicate that telomere length is a good predictor of health and lifespan. Newborns for instance, have telomeres that range in length from 8,000 to 14,000 base pairs. This number declines every year, and by the time someone reaches middle age, they've lost thousands of base pairs from their telomeres.

I'm a big proponent of maintaining telomere length. It is a good biomarker of health. Telomere length testing can be done through a simple blood test. When the test was first was available to the public, it was very expensive, so it was not commonly done; however the price has come down recently, making it more affordable.

I started my age-management program in 2008 and was able to bring down my percent of body fat from 21 percent to 6.7 percent. In 2008, telomere testing was only being done in special research labs and was not readily available. I obtained my first telomere test in 2012, four years into my program. My chronologic age at the time was fifty-eight years. My biologic age, as measured by mean telomere length, showed a biologic age of thirty-nine years. I essentially had the mean telomere length of a thirty-nine year old.

Shortly following that test, I formulated and began taking my own proprietary multivitamin called *Vitamere Ultra Anti Aging*, which was specifically designed to promote DNA health and telomere length. I have been taking Vitamere Ultra ever since. Nothing else has otherwise changed in my age-management program. It has been very consistent. In 2014, I repeated my telomere test. My biological age this time was equal to that of a ten-year-old while my chronologic age was that of a sixty-year-old, an unbelievable fifty-year difference. I didn't believe it at the time, so I ignored it. I repeated my telomere test in May 2017. My chronologic age this time was sixty-two years, but my biologic age, as measured by mean telomere length, was less than that of a twenty year old. The scale ended at age twenty. I was off the scale. When I extrapolated the result, my biological age was that of a twelve year old. This most recent test confirmed that my 2014 telomere test was, in fact, accurate. Wow! What a dramatic improvement in mean telomere length and biological age. Needless to say, I was very happy with the results. My program is producing the kind of results for me that I had hoped for.

Just recently my thirty-two-year-old son who tries to eat sensibly and exercise regularly had his telomeres tested. His results showed a biologic age of twenty-six years. While this is an excellent result, I remain younger than my son at least in biologic telomere years. How is that even possible? How does a father become younger than his son, who is himself younger in telomere years than his chronologic age? I literally have been able to reverse aging by a massive amount—cellular biologic aging that is, as measured by mean telomere length.

I am living proof that telomere shortening can be reversed. A decadent lifestyle with poor eating habits, cigarette smoking, lack of exercise, alcohol, and so forth will shorten your telomeres. A healthy lifestyle with proper eating habits, exercise, and nutritional supplementation can lengthen your telomeres.

When I first began this journey to turn back time and reclaim my life and energy, I was tired, unhealthy, and out of shape. Today I am in the best shape of my life. This is because I made a commitment to take control of my health.

Many people don't know what to do to be healthy. Good health doesn't happen by accident. You have to pay attention. You have to get involved. If you want to get healthy and stay healthy, don't do what sick people do. Develop your own healthy habits and stick to them. You have to be proactive to reduce inflammation, the root cause of chronic disease.

For optimal results in life or in business you need optimal health. Your health is the most important asset you have. Without good health, nothing else really matters. Invest in your health, and make the time to turn things around. If you take your health seriously, you can live feeling younger today than you did twenty years ago.

It's been my experience that most people don't make their health a priority. They take their health for granted until it is too late, and then they want a quick fix. But it doesn't work that way. Just look at any nursing home and you will see the results of that kind of thinking. You can't abuse your body for decades and expect a smooth landing. In contrast, have you ever seen someone who seems to be perpetually joyful and smiling, having a youthful exuberance about them? These are the rare people who stay forever young. They've got an attitude of joy and gratitude that feels contagious! They appear stress free.

Stress can age you. Just look at the pictures of any American president at the start of their term and compare them to their pictures after their term is up. The change is unmistakable. Over the course of history, the media has reported on the way the presidents of the United States age by posting their before and after photos. Wow, what a difference! Search these photos online and you can visibly see the cost of having the highest position in the nation. It ages you. Managing stress is an important age management tool. How's your mindset?

The National Institute of Health (NIH) reports, "Scientists found that age related damage to DNA and proteins is often reversible." In their online article dated November 2011, the NIH stated that "[r]esearchers are studying the relationship between psychological stress and aging. In one study, mothers of severely and chronically sick children had shorter telomeres than other women."

There is no doubt that stress and depression can negatively impact someone's health. Depression is sometimes a result of hormonal deficiencies or imbalance. Patients are sometimes surprised to learn that there are biologic causes of emotional stress and depression. They are not only caused by external events. Maintaining hormones at normal youthful levels and in balance can often reverse many cases of depression and help people manage external stress better.

STRESS IS A CAUSE OF MANY MAJOR DISEASES, INCLUDING STROKE AND HEART ATTACK. STRESS CAN SHORTEN TELOMERES.

Often patients come to us, not realizing that they have hormonal deficiencies or nutritional imbalances causing their sadness, emotional tension, confusion, loss of energy, poor physical health, sexual dysfunction, and even chronic stress. Once we evaluate them and measure their hormone levels, they can begin the journey to solve these issues and attack the problems that prevent them from being productive every day of their life.

Breakthrough advances in anti-aging medicine are showing us that while our chronological age may be inevitable, the visible, mental, and physical aspects of aging are not.

One of the things we do in the anti-aging practice is begin with a complete health evaluation so that we can create a customized program geared to the individual needs of the patient. Many of our patients indicate that our Executive Health Evaluation is the most extensive health assessment they have ever received. We help people understand the biology of aging and how each of these different factors, such as inflammation and telomeres, impact lifestyle.

IF YOU ARE NOT EXPERIENCING THE BEST THAT LIFE HAS TO OFFER IN EVERY AREA— PHYSICAL, MENTAL AND SEXUAL—NOW IS THE TIME TO MAKE A CHANGE.

It is never too early or too late to improve your life in these important areas:

- Physical strength, fitness, and endurance
- Memory, focus, and recall
- Sexual health
- Mood and sense of well-being
- Disease prevention

Overcoming medical challenges like heart disease, obesity, diabetes, osteoporosis, and other aging-related diseases takes intentionality. When you change your mindset to prevention, you're able to attack aging rather than letting it attack you. Alzheimer's is a perfect example of a brain-aging disease that can be potentially prevented with a focus on improving circulation, nutrition, and adopting healthy lifestyle habits.

I became a doctor because I wanted to help sick people. That's still true today, but now I also want to help prevent people from getting sick in the first place. It is a big part of age management.

Medicine is one of the most demanding careers you can have because you can't make a mistake, especially when you're a neurosurgeon. Managing stress is important for anyone in the health care profession in order to provide the best possible care for the patient. I focus on stress management for my mind and body by continually making sure I have the proper nutrition, physical activity, and mindset.

What you do for a career is a large part of your mindset. Everyone has to do something in life and when you're living your passion and doing the job that you feel is your life's purpose, your mindset will be incredibly positive.

If you don't feel you are in the right position or line of work, make a change today! Your mindset will change!

America is a wonderful country, full of opportunities that you just don't have anywhere else. I was born in the Ukraine in a city called Odessa, which the city of Odessa in Texas is named after. I was born in1954 and had an older sister—years older. We lived in a one-room apartment because after the communists took over they basically nationalized everything, and they took people's apartments and put multiple families in one apartment. We literally lived in one room of the apartment.

Imagine that!

You don't have to because chances are you live in America.

When I was growing up, families would have one room that was yours and then you'd share the kitchen or the bathroom down the hall. So, there were four of us literally in one room in our "home" in Russia. My father was a tailor, and he moved us to Poland, his homeland, when I was two. How did I get here, to practice medicine and age management and write these words to you?

My father was Polish and my mother was Russian, and Khrushchev at that time was allowing the Polish Jews and anyone who was Polish who had fled to Russia during World War II to escape the Germans to go back to Poland. We went back to Poland and lived in a town called the Legnica. We shared the bathroom and kitchen with another family, but it was better than before as we now had two rooms instead of one for the four of us and we lived there for about three years. I had an uncle in Paris, France, so we moved from Poland to Paris, and that's where I started first grade. My uncle there owned a small hotel and bed and breakfast so we rented a room from him, and once again the four of us were living in a one-room dwelling. But we were very lucky as we had escaped communism.

Living in all these different countries meant that I had to learn new languages. I first spoke Russian, then Polish, and then French. When I was eight, we had an uncle in the Bronx in New York City who sponsored us, so we emigrated to New York City in 1962.

Moving to New York meant learning english. Within two weeks, I learned English through sign language and picture books. By the time I was nine years old, I spoke five languages fluently: Russian, Polish, English, French, and sign language. My father found work in the garment district, and I went to public school. Once I reached high school age, I tested for the Bronx Science High School, which was a nationally prestigious high school with eight Nobel Laureate graduates, the most of any high schools in the country.

At that school I worked hard, and I was in the top third of the class and then I went to NYU on scholarship. My story—an immigrant who came to America and worked hard for the dream— is available to many. It's the story of many! It was hard work, perseverance, and a determined and positive mindset that got me where I am today! What if I had a negative mindset instead? My parents weren't rich. In fact, we were outright poor. I didn't have anything handed to me. I just worked hard and remained focused and determined.

In college I found out about a program at the Johns Hopkins Unversity School of Medicine called the 2 /5 program, where you apply to medical school at the end of your first year of college or beginning your second year of college. If you were accepted, you would go to Johns Hopkins for five more years, receiving a bachelor's degree after the first year and your doctorate degree four years later, essentially doing college in three years rather than four. They accepted only twelve kids in the country for that program, and guess who made it. That's right. Me.

I attended Hopkins for the following five years, and I got my bachelor's degree in human biology in 1976 from Hopkins and then my medical degree in 1979, also from Hopkins. That was followed by my internship in general surgery at UT Southwestern Medical Center in Dallas at Parkland Hospital and then a five-year residency in neurosurgery at Parkland. I spent a year in London, England, at Queen's Square doing neurosurgery. When I finished my residency in 1985, I moved twenty minutes west to Arlington, Texas, where I've been practicing neurosurgery ever since. Of course, over the past several decades, I discovered that you're only as young as your vascular system! Neurosurgery is a fantastic foundation for age management because you truly get to see the entire picture. What you do to your body affects your brain, and what you do to your brain affects your body. So you really need to look at the whole person.

I've seen the physical side of successful aging and also the mental side. You can be in the best physical shape of your life, but if you don't have the right mindset you can be at risk. What's your perception of the world? Do you feel like a victim, or do you feel as if each day is a gift? Are you living and working with passion and purpose? Do you have the energy to fulfil your dreams?

I have been doing neurosurgery and age management now for a long time and I'm still as enthusiastic about what I'm doing now as I was when I first started many years ago. It's still fascinating, still fun, and still challenging.

My parents were both garment workers who did tailoring in the garment district in New York City. Neither one went to college! They didn't even finish high school because of World War II.

They taught me the value of hard work, discipline, and especially self-reliance.

My father had started working when he was thirteen, and that lesson of hard work wasn't lost on me. I also started working when I was thirteen, delivering meat for a butcher shop just working for tips, and I have been working ever since. When I was young I didn't get an allowance, and I have always known the value of working hard. Mindset is everything, and mindset will get you where you want to go. So don't be afraid to take your first step. Take control of your health now!

Age-intervention medicine is a paradigm shift. Rather than conventional medicine's reactive approach with a focus on symptoms and disease, our proactive approach at the SciLife Southwest Age Intervention Institute uses an integrated and functional approach attacking the root causes. We are not focused on putting out fires. We are focused on preventing them.

CHAPTER 2

THE BIOLOGY
OF AGING

What Is Aging?

Aging is a biologic process of physical and mental changes that gradually occur as we get older. It is a gradual decline of function of the human body over time. Most people don't understand it and are unsure if anything can even be done about it.

To the average person, aging seems like a mystery. They expect not only to get old but to feel old. They expect that the development of chronic disease is inevitable. They expect their energy levels will decline as well as their level of function, both physically and mentally, not to mention sexually. The good news is that it doesn't have to be that way.

Once we understand the biology of aging, we can focus on prevention. There are certain things that occur in aging that we can do something about and others that we can't. We focus on those things that we can influence. Our goal is to delay or prevent the onset of chronic disease and of frailty and feebleness and in the process, reverse aging—at least as can be measured by biomarkers such as mean telomere length.

Aging is the gradual decay of the human body over time. It starts in our cells, spreads to our organs, and then to our bodies.

One of the theories of aging is that over time, damage occurs to our DNA that can't be corrected, which affects protein production, the general function of the cell and ultimately the organ. DNA damage can even cause cancer. So, taking good care of our DNA through healthy lifestyle habits and supportive nutritional supplements is important if we want to extend our health span. My *Vitamere Anti Aging* and *Vitamere Ultra Anti Aging Supplements Multivitamins* are specifically formulated to support DNA health.

Another theory of aging is the gradual shortening of our telomeres over time. As previously mentioned, telomeres are our cellular timekeepers. They make up the ends of our DNA. They keep the DNA from unraveling. When telomeres get too short, the cell is no longer able to divide.

I'M AN ANTI-AGING ADVOCATE WHO FOCUSES ON HEALTH AND WELLNESS BECAUSE I'VE SEEN WHAT HAPPENS TO UNHEALTHY PEOPLE AND THE DAMAGE THEY DO TO THEMSELVES

The longer your telomeres are, the younger your cells are and the younger you are in terms of biologic age. Telomere length has been used as a marker of biologic age. There are several scientific studies and articles that indicate that telomere length is a good predictor of lifespan. So, you want to keep your telomeres as long as possible. If you start an intervention, such as an age-management or anti-aging program, or start a supplement specifically formulated to support telomere length, and your mean telomere length increases as a result of this intervention, you have essentially reversed cellular aging. We now have a way to measure this, so you can see if what you are doing is working or not.

As I mentioned earlier, I was able to increase my mean telomere length from that of a thirty-nine year old in 2012 to that of a twenty year old in May 2017. I started my age-management, anti-aging program in 2008. In 2008, mean telomere length testing was not available outside of the experimental lab setting, and I was not aware of its availability. Between 2008 and 2012, I took a standard multivitamin as part of my age-management program.

In 2012, I began taking *Vitamere Ultra*, a proprietary multivitamin I developed that not only has the normal vitamins, minerals, and trace elements of a regular multivitamin, but it also contains ingredients that in the scientific literature were shown to support telomere length. In 2012 before taking *Vitamere Ultra*, my chronologic age was fifty-eight years and my biologic age was thirty-nine years, as measured by mean telomere length. I thought that was pretty good until May 2017 when I repeated my telomere testing after taking *Vitamere Ultra Anti Aging Multivitamins* for five years.

At this point my chronologic age was sixty-two years but my biologic age was an amazing twenty years as measured by mean telomere length. In fact, it was that of someone younger than age twenty as the scale ended at twenty years and I was off of the scale. Extrapolating, my mean telomere length was actually that of a twelve year old. The only difference between what I was doing before 2012 and after 2012 was taking *Vitamere Ultra Anti Aging Multivitamins*. Nothing else had changed in my age-management program. It was otherwise identical before and after 2012.

Now that's a quick overview on some of the biology of aging. For the average patient, the only thing they really understand is that they begin to feel the symptoms of aging after a walk up a flight of stairs, after an injury that's difficult to rebound from, or when their performance physically or sexually isn't what it used to be.

To understand *why* this all happens, however, it's important to understand the human body and how we can make positive choices and changes that can potentially reverse the damage.

Nutrition and Your Body

Foods can affect gene expression. The study of this phenomenon is known as *nutrigenomics*.

In the twentieth century, nutritional science focused on finding vitamin and minerals to prevent deficiency diseases and to promote health focused on epidemiology and physiology.

In the twenty-first century, the focus of nutritional science and research has shifted into looking at how nutrients act at the molecular and gene level. In nutrigenomics, nutrients are cell signals, which interact with genes and protein expression and thus affect cellular metabolism and function. In nutrigenomics, we try to find nutritional supplements and bioactive food compounds that can have a positive effect on health.

FOOD IS MEDICINE, WHICH MEANS THAT YOU HAVE FAR MORE CONTROL OVER YOUR HEALTH THAN YOU EVER THOUGHT POSSIBLE!

An example of the application of nutrigenomics is the reversal of cellular aging as measured by telomere length. Anything that can maintain telomere length or rebuild telomere length will enable the cell to keep replicating, thus prolonging the life of the cell and potentially the organism. In theory, the cell would never get old and die.

Reverse Aging Today

As studies of centenarians have shown, the length of a person's telomeres is a good indicator of overall health. Short telomeres have been associated with accelerated cellular aging and dysfunction. To maintain good health, it is important to maintain telomere length. Having short telomeres can accelerate the natural aging process on a cellular level. Thus, to remain healthy and slow down cellular aging and the aging process in general, you must maintain the length of your telomeres. A good place to start is with the adaptation of healthier lifestyle habits such as exercise, proper nutrition, weight loss, and smoking cessation.

Take appropriate nutritional supplements! Supplementation is important to fill the gaps in our imperfect diet. With the introduction of *Vitamere* and *Vitamere Ultra Anti Aging Multivitamins* in our supplementation program in my age-management practice, individuals take advantage of the most recent research in nutrigenomics by taking these supplements, which can support their telomeres with nutraceuticals specifically designed for this purpose.

Not only are we meeting our general health needs with a broad spectrum, high-potency multivitamin/mineral formula containing all the essential vitamins, minerals, and trace elements that we need, but we are getting additional ingredients, including antioxidants and phytonutrients to help protect our DNA and extend the life of our telomeres.

When aging occurs, the body decays. Why and how does it specifically decay? To start, let's look at our organs. While we are born with normal, healthy organs, they eventually begin to lose function over time, and the rate of that function loss can depend on your health habits and lifestyle. How well do you take care of yourself, and what do you put into your body? Organs can be impacted by chemicals, toxins, alcohol, and sugar.

YOUR LIFESTYLE HABITS WILL DETERMINE THE HEALTH OF YOUR BLOOD VESSELS.

Although each organ is different, they all have one very important thing in common: they all need excellent blood flow to deliver nutrients and oxygen and remove waste. Without proper blood flow, the organ cannot do its job, and its cells cannot repair any damage produced because of normal metabolism and oxidative stress. As the cells get sick and old, so does the organ. If blood flow stops, the organ dies. Poor blood flow will lead to accelerated aging. We are only as healthy as our blood vessels.

That's just one of the explanations of how we age. Another is *oxidative stress*.

Biological stress occurs constantly from everyday metabolic activity. When you eat food and breathe in oxygen, the body utilizes glucose by combining it with oxygen to produce energy—which is metabolism. This metabolic reaction produces free radicals, which must be neutralized by antioxidants or cell damage will occur. The more free radicals, the more antioxidants you need to neutralize them. Extreme physical exertion, such as running a marathon for instance, can create so many free radicals that they overwhelm the body's ability to neutralize them, potentially causing damage to your body. Yet running by itself can keep you fit and healthy if you don't overdo it.

You can help fight oxidative stress by eating foods rich in antioxidants and phytonutrients. These are typically very colorful fruits and vegetables, such as blueberries, raspberries, blackberries, strawberries, carrots, and bell peppers to mention a few. Fruits and vegetables that are purple, red, blue, orange, and yellow typically are rich in antioxidants.

There's an ongoing debate about the value of supplements to your overall health, but there's no denying that your body needs key nutrients, including antioxidants such as vitamins A, C, D, and E, in order to survive and thrive.

It amazes me how many patients who come to see me are vitamin D deficient. Over 90 percent are suboptimal in their vitamin D levels. A significant number are also suboptimal in vitamin B12, which is essential for energy production and overall well-being.

Vitamin deficiencies can lead to serious health issues but are easy to prevent simply by eating a healthy diet with a lot of fruits and vegetables and supplementing with multivitamins to fill in any holes in your diet. How do we balance and maintain health and fitness? The key is to understand and harness the knowledge of the biology of aging. Only then can we put into action a strategic plan to extend your health and lifespan. It's important to note that I don't want to extend your life span only. It's about extending your health span. It's about keeping you healthy and energetic for as long as possible. No one cheats death, but you can extend your life and live each day with vigor, vitality, and boundless energy! This is very possible, and it's a reality for many of my patients.

You extend your life by avoiding the things that shorten your life. It really is as simple as that, and I want to show you how. This is critically important for most people to understand sooner rather than later. Most people have so many misconceptions about health that they're actually doing the wrong things. I know a guy who is overweight who decided to eat lots of fruit and drink a lot of juices to lose weight.

It may have been slightly better than his previous diet of fast food, yet fruit and fruit juice are loaded with sugar, and he wasn't losing weight. Many people I encounter also have misconceptions about the way the brain ages and resort to a lot of things that aren't going to help their brain. The brain is simply an organ, a part of your body. You've got to take care of it!

CIRCULATION AND BLOOD FLOW ARE ABSOLUTELY CRITICAL TO BRAIN HEALTH AND FUNCTION. THIS IS WHERE EXERCISE PLAYS A ROLE.

Most people begin to see the evidence of aging in their skin and start fighting it by covering it up instead of getting at the root cause. When they get wrinkles, they may go on to get Botox. When their skin gets dry, they cover it up with moisturizer. What they don't realize is that they are getting older on the inside as well, but they can't see it. They can only feel it. The way to get healthy, youthful-looking skin is from the inside out. Circulation, circulation, circulation. How do you get that? You get it by momentum. You cannot be sedentary and live a long and healthy life. If you know someone who sits on the couch every night, glued to the television set, chances are they aren't going to live as long or as healthy as they could.

You've probably heard some people say things like, "My grandfather didn't exercise and lived to be eighty!" The next time someone says things like that, you may want to ask how well their grandfather got around, whether he was in a wheelchair or took long walks and enjoyed traveling the world. It's one thing to live to eighty and quite another to live a healthy life with boundless energy.

Aging starts early, and often we just don't notice, or we attribute it to a temporary situation and try to fix it with temporary solutions.

The signs and symptoms of aging, such as thin, dry, and fragile skin, loss of muscle mass, cognitive decline, diminished libido, diminished sexual function, and lack of energy and zest for life, come on gradually. By the time you notice these changes, things have deteriorated internally to a significant degree, but you attribute them to normal aging and as inevitable. You don't realize that there are things that you can do to feel better and reverse a lot of these symptoms. I'm in my sixties, and I've got more energy now than I did in my twenties and thirties. I'm living proof that it doesn't have to be that way. You don't have to feel old as you get old. People may look at my before and after pictures and come up with a myriad of excuses as to why they can't achieve that, but I'm here to tell you that you can. I turned back the hands of time and so can you. If a busy neurosurgeon who is constantly seeing patients and doing complicated surgeries daily can still work out every day, what's stopping you?

This isn't brain surgery. The truth is you have the power to change your life.

Once you get your blood tested, begin measuring your biomarkers and stats, and you will discover the truth about what is really going on in your body. Then you will be able to make the changes required to optimize your health. You will have a baseline from which you will be able to tell if what you are doing is working or not. By regularly monitoring and measuring your biomarkers, you will be able tell if you are going off track or not. You can then make adjustments before things get really out of control. The secret is to be aware of negative trends early before they do their damage. In my anti-aging practice, I help people take back their life again! We give them a new lease on life filled with energy so that they can live better, healthier, and stronger than ever before. Of course, when we understand the biology of aging from the inside out, we can see that it's an inside job that begins with nutrition. How we appear on the outside is directly related to what we put into our bodies and the effect it has on what is happening on the inside.

Want to grow your hair, or look better and have softer, thicker, more velvety skin? Focus on making better food choices, and you'll begin to see immediate changes in the way you look. Have you ever seen one of those weight loss shows, such as *The Biggest Loser*? Often, it's hard to tell who the person is after the weight loss because they appear so different. When you see the after picture, it's hard to imagine that it was the same person they featured in the before segment! When people make a commitment to change, everything transforms, and it can be quite astonishing. My own before and after photos are evidence of a profound transformation both inside my body metabolically and outside physically. How you appear on the outside can give us good clues as to what might be happening on the inside.

PREVENTING OXIDATIVE STRESS AND INFLAMMATION WILL HELP YOU AGE WELL

As you read through these pages, you'll see that I'm focused on a healthy body from the inside out. I often say to my patients, "You're only as healthy as your blood vessels."

It has been estimated that you have about 100,000 miles of blood vessels in your body if you connected them end to end. If they're not healthy, you can't deliver oxygen and nutrients to your cells or take away waste. You can't attain peak performance. My

focus is to make sure you are equipped with the right information, so you can make the best possible decisions to impact your
health positively, both inside and out. If your arteries are clear,
your body and mind are functioning at their best. By exercising
and eating right, you'll feel better and live longer.

A healthy life really is that simple.

CHAPTER 3

THE DISAPPEARING SKINNY

Society is getting fatter and fatter, so much so that skinny is becoming extinct.

Yes, that's right. Skinny people, as defined as people with a normal body mass index (BMI 18.5–24.9), a reasonable definition in today's world, are becoming extinct! If you don't believe me, here are the stats. According to the Centers for Disease Control and Prevention National Center for Health Statistics (CDC), in 2013–2014, the percent of adults age twenty years and over who were obese was 37.9 percent (BMI 30 or >). Another 32.8 percent of adults were overweight (BMI 25–29.9). Only 29.3 percent had a normal BMI. It is frightening to think that 70.7 percent of the adult population is either overweight or obese. Putting this in round numbers, more than two-thirds of our population is either overweight or obese. Less than one-third is skinny, what we are calling people with normal BMI in this chapter. A whopping 40 percent (in round numbers) is obese, the largest segment of our population.

These numbers are getting worse over time. According to the CDC, the prevalence of obesity increased between 1999 and 2014, going from 30.5 percent to almost 38 percent.

But it's not only adults who are getting fat; obesity is prevalent in our children and adolescents as well. The older our children get, the greater the incidence of obesity has become. Here are the numbers for 2013–2014 from a CDC report:

- Percent of adolescents age 12–19 years with obesity: 20.6 percent

- Percent of children age 6–11 years with obesity: 17.4 percent

- Percent of children age 2–5 years with obesity: 9.4 percent

Imagine being five or six years old and being obese! How can that happen? But the facts show that about one in ten children two to five years of age is obese, as is one in five adolescents. Our modern way of life is not consistent with good health and wellness. No wonder we spend so much on healthcare. Rather than get at the root cause of illness, we spend our healthcare dollars on treating the symptoms.

INSTEAD OF TRYING TO PUT OUT FIRES, WE SHOULD FOCUS ON PREVENTING THE FIRE FROM STARTING IN THE FIRST PLACE.

The statistics look even worse if we look at the diabetic population, 95 percent of whom are type 2 diabetics. Type 2 diabetics do not respond to insulin. They make insulin, but their bodies are resistant to it. Type 2 diabetes is usually the result of poor diet and lifestyle habits. In Type 1 diabetes, the body does not make enough insulin. It is believed to be caused by an autoimmune reaction where the body attacks its own insulin-producing cells in the pancreas. There is no known way to prevent or reverse type 1 diabetes. Type 2 diabetes is preventable and can be reversed with diet, weight loss, and proper lifestyle habits.

According to the CDC, nearly half of adult Americans have diabetes or prediabetes. The numbers are staggering. Thirty million Americans have diabetes, which represents 12.2 percent of all US adults. Of these, almost 25 percent do not even know they have it.

For prediabetes, the statistics are even worse. Eighty-four million adult Americans are prediabetic, which represents 34 percent of the adult population. Of these, 9 out of 10 don't know they are prediabetic. Combined, the incidence of diabetes and prediabetes is 46.1 percent or almost half of all adult Americans. Fifteen to 30 percent of people with prediabetes will develop type 2 diabetes within 5 years.

How would you know if you're prediabetic? The bad news is that many people don't. Many people ignore symptoms and keep on trudging through life until it's too late.

As the population ages, the incidence of diabetes gets even worse. Almost three-fourths of adults age 65 or greater are diabetic or prediabetic. (25.2 percent are diabetic and 48.3 percent are prediabetic.) This does not bode well for longevity because diabetics have a risk of death 50 percent higher than nondiabetics. Diabetes is the seventh-leading cause of death, but this number is probably understated, as diabetes is not always listed on death certificates.

From the economic perspective, diabetes is a drain on our wallets and our economy. Medical costs for diabetics are twice that of nondiabetics. The cost of diagnosed diabetics in the United States in 2012 was estimated at $245 billion in both medical costs and lost work and wages. This number can easily double to almost half a trillion dollars if 30 percent of today's prediabetics go on to become diabetic, as the statistics suggest that 15–30 percent of prediabetics go on to become diabetic.

If we look at BMI in diabetics, skinny is becoming even more extinct in this population. According to a 2017 CDC report, 87.5 percent of diabetics are either obese or overweight. Only 12.5 percent have a normal BMI. The breakdown is as follows:

- 26.1 percent overweight (BMI 25–29.9)
- 43.5 percent obese (BMI 30–39.9)
- 17.8 percent severe obesity (BMI 40 & >)
- 12.5 percent normal BMI (BMI <25)

People ask me, "Why to do you want to be skinny and deprive yourself of all those wonderful sweets and sugary food?" And the answer is because it is healthier than being fat. If being fat was healthy there would nothing wrong with being fat. *In fact, if being fat was healthier than being skinny, then I would be fat because I want to do everything that I can to stay as healthy as I can.* But this is not the case. Obesity and being overweight are not good for your health. People who are overweight or obese are much more likely to get diabetes, cancer, and cardiovascular disease, including strokes and heart attacks, compared to normal-weight adults. Their mortality rates are increased. The higher your BMI, the greater your all-cause mortality rate.

When you look at the facts, it makes you pay attention.

A recent study showed that about one in five deaths is linked to people being overweight or obese (Ryan Masters PhD, et al., *American Journal of Public Health*, 8/15/13). In this study 18.2 percent of all deaths in adults ages 40 to 85 between 1986 and 2006 were associated with their being overweight or obese. The more recent their year of birth, the more likely obesity played a role. We are seeing obesity in younger and younger people, which exposes them to the deleterious effects of obesity (chronic diseases) for longer periods of time during their lifetime, thus affecting them more. The risk of obesity affecting mortality increases with increasing age. Obesity is threatening to reverse the steady increase in life expectancy we have seen over the past hundred years.

A large study was done by the Global BMI Mortality Collaboration comprised of five hundred investigators from three hundred worldwide institutions looking at the association between excess body weight as determined by BMI and premature death (*Lancet*

2016; 388:776–86). They analyzed 4 million adults who were followed for an average of 14 years. People with normal BMI had the lowest mortality risk. The risk of dying increased significantly as the BMI increased:

- BMI 26–<27.5: 7 percent higher risk of mortality
- BMI 27.5–<30: 20 percent higher risk of mortality
- BMI 30–<35.0: 45 percent higher risk of mortality
- BMI 35–<40.0: 94 percent higher risk of mortality
- BMI 40–<60.0: 292 percent higher risk of mortality

For every 5-unit increase in BMI above 25, there was about a 31 percent increased risk of dying.

When they looked at the specific causes of death, for each 5-unit increase in BMI above 25, there was a 49 percent increase in cardiovascular deaths, a 38 percent increase in respiratory disease–related deaths, and a 19 percent increase in cancer-related deaths.

Many studies have shown that increased BMI is associated with an increased prevalence of type 2 diabetes, high blood pressure, elevated cholesterol, and cancer. As our society gets fatter and fatter, we are getting sicker and sicker. The fatter we get, the shorter we live. We are at the point where our children's life expectancy may be less than ours if these trends continue because children are getting fatter at a younger age and thus exposed to chronic disease for a longer percentage of their lifetime than previous generations.

CHAPTER 4

DNA AND TELOMERES

All human behavior is governed by the interaction of various neuro-humoral pathways and relays, all of which are determined by our DNA. Our DNA ultimately is responsible for who we are, what we are, and our behavior. DNA gave us our frontal lobes for judgment, so we can control our primitive reptilian brain and make smart decisions.

DNA wants to propel itself into the future in a more resilient and survivable form. It is designed for this by its capacity to change so as to be better able to adapt to its ever-changing environment. It is always trying to make itself better. This is called evolution. Reproduction is all about this. DNA contains our genes. Some genes are good; others are bad. It depends on the environment that they find themselves in.

While DNA may load the gun, environment pulls the trigger. What this means is that even if you have bad genes, such as genes predisposing you to cancer, it doesn't mean you will inevitably get cancer. A lot of this is related to your environment. If you adopt healthy lifestyle habits, including eating lots of colorful vegetables and fruits, exercise, and avoiding smoking, you may never get cancer as you are surrounding yourself with a healthy environment. On the other hand, if you smoke, eat poorly, and never exercise, you are setting yourself up for poor health and may very well end up getting cancer, especially if you are genetically predisposed to it. Food can turn off bad genes and turn on good genes. It all depends on your lifestyle. Food can be medicine, or food can be a poison. It's up to you what you make it. It's up to you what you will place in your mouth.

To keep your brain healthy, challenge it, but also supply it with the proper nutrients to keep it healthy and give it the ability to fight off free radicals, oxidative stress, and inflammation because that's how you combat brain diseases. If you don't challenge yourself, then you won't grow. If you don't eat right and supplement correctly, you will be depriving your brain and your body of vital nutrients.

Does DNA Matter?

The answer is that of course it matters, but don't place so much emphasis on it that you think it matters too much.

While your DNA matters and plays a vital role in how healthy you may be, environment is just as important. Therefore, prevention and lifestyle are just as critical to your overall health, wellness, and longevity. How you live each day determines how well you age.

Your brain function doesn't have to decline as it may have in your ancestors. If your grandmother had dementia, it doesn't mean you will, too. If I had a dollar for every human I heard tell me that their grandfather ate junk food and lived to be ninety, I'd be a millionaire. It doesn't matter if your grandfather ate fried chicken and donuts and lived to old age. Maybe he was lucky. Maybe you won't be so lucky! The point is, make smart choices when it comes to your health. Don't play roulette with your health.

Cells make up the basic building blocks of all living things. The human body is composed of trillions of cells, which make up all of our organs. Each cell contains a nucleus, which acts as the cell's command center. It directs all cell function, which includes the making of proteins, cell division, growth, maturation, and death.

The nucleus contains our DNA (deoxyribonucleic acid), the hereditary material in all organisms. The information in DNA is stored as a code made of up four chemical bases: adenine (A), guanine (G), cytosine (C), and thymine (T). Human DNA contains about 3 billion bases, 99 percent of which are the same in everyone. The remaining 1 percent differs slightly and is responsible for our uniqueness.

The sequence of these bases determines the building and maintenance of the organism. It determines who we are, what we look like, and how we function.

DNA bases pair up with each other (A with T and C with G) to form units called base pairs. Each base is also attached to a sugar molecule and a phosphate molecule. The unit consisting of a base, a sugar molecule, and a phosphate molecule is called a nucleotide. Nucleotides are arranged in two long strands that form a spiral called a double helix.

A unique function of DNA is the ability to replicate itself and make exact copies of itself. Each strand of the double helix in DNA serves as a pattern for duplicating the sequences of bases.

DNA contains our genes, the basic unit of heredity. Genes give instructions to our cells to make substances known as proteins. Genes vary in size from a few hundred DNA bases to more than 2 million bases.

Humans have between 20,000 and 25,000 genes. Each person has 2 copies of each gene, one inherited from their father, the other from their mother. Most genes are the same in everyone, but a small number of genes (less than 1 percent) are slightly different in their sequence. These minor differences are responsible for each person's uniqueness and difference in physical characteristics.

Gene expression can be turned on and off in a cell. Each cell turns on only a fraction of its genes. The remainder remain turned off (are repressed). This is known as gene regulation.

Chemical compounds that are added to single genes can regulate a gene's activity. These changes are known as epigenetic changes. These compounds are not part of the DNA sequence but are attached to the DNA. They can be inherited and are influenced by environmental factors, such as pollution, diet, exercise, food, and nutrients. They can turn genes on and off.

DNA is packaged in a cell nucleus into threadlike structures known as chromosomes. In humans, each cell normally contains twenty-three pairs of chromosomes for a total of forty-six chromosomes. Twenty-two of these pairs look the same in both males and females. The twenty-third pair contains the two sex chromosomes, which are different in males and females. Females have two copies of the X chromosome, one from each parent. Males have one X chromosome from the mother and one Y chromosome from the father; thus the father determines the sex of the offspring.

All of this may sound like mumbo jumbo to you, but if you study it like I have, it makes a lot of sense. The choices you make with your diet impact how long you'll live. You can impact your body chemistry and hormones by adding supplements and making the right daily activity and food choices.

Why Is Food So Critical?

Foods can affect gene expression. The study of this phenomenon is known as nutrigenomics. In the twentieth century, nutritional science focused on finding vitamin and minerals to prevent deficiency diseases and promote health focused on epidemiology and physiology.

In the twenty-first century, the focus of nutritional science and research has shifted into looking at how nutrients act at the molecular and gene level. In nutrigenomics, nutrients are cell signals, which interact with genes and protein expression and thus affect cellular metabolism and function.

In nutrigenomics, we try to find nutritional supplements and bioactive food compounds that can have a positive effect on health. An example of the application of nutrigenomics is the reversal of cellular aging as measured by mean telomere length.

Anything that can maintain telomere length or rebuild telomere length will enable the cell to keep replicating, thus prolonging the life of the cell and potentially the organism. In theory, the cell would never get old and die. The length of a person's telomeres is a good indicator of overall health. To maintain good health, it is important to maintain telomere length. Having short telomeres can accelerate the natural aging process on a cellular level.

A good place to start is with the adaptation of healthier life-style habits, such as exercise, proper nutrition, weight loss, and smoking cessation. You'll hear me repeat this often throughout the book!

With the introduction of *Vitamere Anti Aging* and *Vitamere Ultra Anti Aging*, we can take advantage of the most recent research in nutrigenomics and support our telomeres with nutraceuticals specifically designed for this purpose. Not only are we meeting our general health needs with a broad-spectrum, high-quality, potent multivitamin/mineral formula containing all the essential vitamins, minerals, and trace elements that we need, but we have added additional ingredients, including antioxidants and phyto-nutrients, to help protect and extend the life of your telomeres.

Telomeres Are Your Cellular Time Keepers.

They determine the rate at which you age. The body has a pro-tective enzyme known as telomerase. Telomerase helps to rebuild, protect, repair, and lengthen your telomeres. It was initially be-lieved that once a cell matures and is no longer a stem cell, telo-merase turns off and you can no longer maintain telomeres. It turns out that this is not entirely true.

Recent research shows that there are specific nutrients that stimulate your body to turn on the enzyme telomerase, which helps to rebuild your telomeres. Using this research, we now have a scientifically validated way to support telomeres so that they remain longer for a longer period of time, thus maintaining and even reversing cellular aging as defined by mean telomere length.

The ingredients in *Vitamere Anti Aging* and *Vitamere Ultra Anti Aging* are supported by combining findings from 402 peer-reviewed scientific studies. These ingredients will help support your telomeres, widely believed to be your cellular time keepers. The longer your telomeres, as measured by mean telomere length, the "younger" your cells and the healthier you are.

But supplementation with *Vitamere Anti Aging* by itself isn't everything and probably not enough. A healthy lifestyle in combination with supplementation is needed for optimal health and maintaining telomere length. I'm a busy surgeon, but I also find the time to exercise six days a week and focus on eating clean. And by clean, I mean *clean!* I allow myself no bread, no sugar, no processed foods, and no refined carbs of any kind, without exceptions.

I CHANGED MY OWN LIFE, AND SO CAN YOU. I'M HERE TO SHOW YOU WHAT REALLY WORKS.

Alcoholic beverages in moderation are acceptable if you limit them to no more than two per day, but I would not recommend that you drink every day. Liquors such as vodka or Scotch add needless calories, while wine adds sugar in addition to calories. So minimizing or abstaining from alcoholic drinks is another healthy habit I've adopted. I can't force my patients (or you!) to adopt these same habits, but if you want to look younger, feel younger, and have a clear brain, you should. Let us not forget that alcohol can be toxic to our brains and our livers. If you don't believe me, just get your blood drawn on a Monday after a weekend of drinking and look at your liver enzymes. You might be shocked at what you find.

Many people don't know what to do to stay healthy. One of the reasons is that they have limited ways of measuring their progress. They end up trying one thing or another but don't stick to a game plan. One of the things we do in our age-management practice is measure body composition on a regular basis with a Lunar iDXA machine. We can measure the exact amount of fat, lean tissue (muscle mass), and bone mass to the gram, not only for your body, but also by body regions such as belly, hips, trunk, legs, arms, and so on. This is far more accurate than BMI in assessing health and body composition. We can monitor very closely how you are progressing in your program. We can tell whether or not you are losing fat or gaining muscle and exactly how much to the gram. Many people can have a normal BMI, which is a calculation based on your height and weight, and still be fat. You can be what is called "skinny fat," a situation where you look skinny, but in reality, you have too much fat and not enough muscle. Too much body fat, even if you look skinny, is not healthy. Body fat is inflammatory. Abdominal fat (also known as visceral fat) is especially inflammatory. It produces and releases inflammatory molecules known as cytokines, which chronically inflame your body. Chronic inflammation is a major cause of chronic disease and aging.

To maintain muscle mass, you must do weight training. To burn fat, you must do cardio. To build muscle, you must also eat protein because protein contains amino acids, the building blocks of muscle. Maintaining adequate and preferably optimal hormone levels are also critical to maintaining a healthy body composition as they help burn fat and build muscle. As we get older, we all tend to lose muscle mass. This is known as age-related sarcopenia. It is one of the causes of feebleness and frailty. Without adequate muscle mass, it is hard to ambulate and keep our balance. This is one of the reasons elderly people are so prone to falling. They lack enough muscle to be able to stabilize their core and maintain balance. Add to this age-related bone loss (osteopenia and osteoporosis), and you have a recipe for disaster. Hip fractures in the elderly can be fatal. Hormones are also extremely important in maintaining bone mass, especially in postmenopausal women.

We want to ensure our patients operate at their best and avoid sarcopenia and osteoporosis. This is why weight resistance training and optimal hormonal balance is so important.

I recommend you exercise six times per week, doing a combination of resistance training and cardio. My routine is one hour of resistance training three times a week alternating with forty-five minutes of cardio three times a week for a total of six days a week. One day I will do cardio, the next day I do weight training, the following day cardio again, and so on. If for some reason I miss a day, I will either double up the next day or make up the workout on my "off" day.

YEAR AFTER YEAR, I SEE PATIENTS AND GIVE THEM ADVICE, BUT UNFORTUNATELY SOMETIMES THEY NEVER TAKE IT.

How does that stack up against what you do daily? It's never too late to start.

Exercise is not hard. It's simple. Proper technique means less weight and full range of motion of your joints and muscle. Many people make the mistake of trying to lift too much weight at the expense of range of motion. They use momentum to move the weight rather than their muscle. It is better to use less weight and take the muscle through a full range of motion. This method will spare your joints as well, which can be damaged if you use excess weight. Many people make weight training programs so much harder than they should be.

The Secret to Living a Long Life Is to Stay Healthy

This statement seems rather obvious, but most people ignore this in their day-to-day lifestyles. They make the wrong choices. Many don't know that there are better, healthier ways to go through life. Others know but perhaps are in denial or too set in their ways. Some people just don't care. This latter category doesn't describe you, however, because if it did you wouldn't be reading this book.

You're reading this book because you've got a passion for improving yourself. Even if you feel as if you're too far behind or you've let yourself go, there's hope on the horizon. Work out daily, and commit to improving your eating habits by adopting a radical regimen. I say radical because it is radical for most people to delete sugar from their diets!

How to Work Out

When you work out, you have to work your whole body. You can concentrate on different body regions on different days, but over the course of a week, you should hit all the major body regions such as chest, arms, back, shoulders, and legs. The elliptical machine and the stair master are excellent for cardio. You can vary speed and resistance to get your heart rate into your target range. I always monitor my heart rate when doing cardio so that I know my workout is effective.

Exercise is excellent for your hormones and mood. All your good hormones, including testosterone and growth hormone, and everything that impacts the brain, including endorphins, your body's natural morphine, are released during exercise, impacting your telomeres and helping to fight the aging process.

There's a difference between life span and health span. It's important to have a healthy life span, rather than just extending your life. That period of time in your life in which you are in optimal health is your health span versus just living a long, frail life. Just because you age doesn't mean you have to get old.

CHAPTER 5

LIFESTYLE CHOICES

Americans are some of the fattest people in the world and, as a result, some of the most inflamed. They eat the wrong things because they are always on the go and simply don't have the discipline to say no to fast and unhealthy food. But ultimately the only one you cheat with a lack of self-control is yourself. Eating the wrong things can make you old fast.

We still don't know everything about the human body. I don't believe we have discovered all of the hormones that are at play in our bodies. We are probably still just scratching the surface. But what we do know is enough to help you reverse the damage of free radicals and age better than ever before. The resources and tools we have at our disposal today are phenomenal and life-changing. We know we want less fat around our midsection and our bodies overall. We know we want more muscle mass, and we know that it takes hard work to get it. The key to living a healthier lifestyle is to develop healthy habits and put to work the knowledge that we do have about the human body. We need to develop a routine. Healthy living needs to become a habit.

The power of habit is exponential. You get back much more than you put in. One of the best ways to develop a habit is to make it a priority. What you make a priority, you will do.

If you haven't yet developed a workout routine, or don't know how, you can hire a personal trainer or watch some videos. You can start on your own by joining a gym and using their weight machines and cardio equipment. Most weight machines come with instructions. You can start with light weight as you learn how to use the machine and how it works and gradually increase the weight, repetitions, and sets. Free weights are also easy to use. If you are not sure, you can always ask for help. Most gyms have personal trainers who can assist you. Your workout doesn't have to be anything fancy. This is the way I started out. The key is to maintain a consistent habit and exercise regularly, preferably six days a week. If you make it a priority, you will do it.

SUCCESSFUL PEOPLE HAVE HABITS INGRAINED IN THEIR DAILY CALENDAR THAT HELP THEM SUCCEED.

Chronic inflammation is at the root of most health issues. By developing a habit of working out and eating right, you will be able to fight it. A sedentary lifestyle merely feeds it. It all comes down to the lifestyle choices you make. If you want to reduce belly fat and want your jeans to fit better, develop a habit of working out regularly. Fat cells (especially belly fat cells) are the building blocks of inflammation.

People can blame health problems on genetics, but genetics merely load the gun. Your lifestyle, environment, and your food and exercise choices are what pull the trigger. We can age well, and we can do it with vigor and vitality. Most people want to live a long, healthy, and functional life. They want a long health span, not merely a long life span. They want to stay healthy and vital for as long as possible.

Let's do this together!

Some diet gurus will try to sell the public on the secrets to weight loss. I see a lot of books with titles like how to lose ten pounds in a week, how to shed ten pounds through fasting or detox, and how to lose weight quickly! Losing weight is essential if you're overweight, but keeping it off requires determination and commitment. It's not about a diet. It's about a change of lifestyle. Diets by themselves don't work in the long term.

Good health requires participation, which requires knowledge. I am here to educate you so you can take control of your health. Hopefully, I've already shown you that excellent health isn't a secret. There's no hidden secret or formula at all. It's about empowering you to make the right choices every single day, and that's exactly what I'm here to do.

The journey of life is the greatest journey you will ever be on, and it continues even after you are gone. Make your mark. Don't waste your time on Earth. I want to encourage you to think of your lifestyle in terms of passing on a health and wellness legacy to others. What mark will you leave behind on this planet? Will you be known as the one who simply cannot get enough energy to get off the couch and play with your grandchildren? Or will your legacy be one that your kids and colleagues remember as one of energetic youth? You've got a choice. Define who you are today, and think about what you'd like your legacy to be.

Lifestyle is a choice, and that means you have to overcome instant gratification and dig in and do the hard work to get the results you want. I learned this early on as a child. I learned that there are no excuses except the ones you create for yourself. It doesn't matter if you weren't taught these things; it's never too late to learn! If you didn't have rich parents who had organic meals delivered to your door like the options we have today, or if you simply didn't learn the value of eating well, now is the time. It's my hope that this book educates and inspires.

Looking and feeling younger is not a quick fix but a consistent lifestyle plan. It's a series of daily habits and choices.

It's not instantaneous kind of thing. You've got to work toward your goal, and you've got to pay your dues. Nothing is given to you, and even though others can provide you with education and knowledge, only you can do the actual work. This lesson came through for me very early on in my life. I learned that even though America is a great country, and that there's a lot of opportunity, you have to execute and make it happen because no one is going to do it for you.

Being a doctor is inspiration enough to stay healthy and focused! As a neurosurgeon you have to think fast on your feet because minutes and even seconds matter.

If you make the right decision, you've saved someone's life, but if you made the wrong decision then you didn't. One patient that comes to mind was a twenty-seven-year-old male transported by ambulance to Parkland Hospital after being involved in a car accident. I was chief resident at the time at Parkland, a level one trauma center. We took care of a lot of head injuries there. He arrived comatose, and his C.T. scan showed a right subdural hematoma (blood clot on the brain). So I took him to surgery and drained the blood clot that was putting pressure on his brain. When we went to wake him up, he had a "blown pupil" on the left side, a sign that there was pressure on the left side of the brain.

The standard protocol would have been to take him to radiology and obtain another C.T. scan to see what was going on. But that takes time, and this patient didn't have time. He was so bad he would have died if I had not made the decision to open up the other side of his head. Sure enough, he had a blood clot that had developed on the left side that wasn't visible on the original scan. When we drained the right-sided blood clot, it had taken the pressure off the left side of the brain that was keeping injured blood vessels from bleeding, and so they bled, creating a new problem on the left side.

We drained the second blood clot immediately and saved his life. The kid did great.

The next day at a staff conference, I was asked, "Why didn't you take him to C.T. scan?" "He would have died," I explained, "There wasn't time for that." Sometimes you have to go with your gut instincts and do what is right rather than what is standard protocol.

That's what I mean by thinking on your feet. Sometimes you have to think faster and a little bit outside the box. You can't always stick to strict protocol. There are times in your life when you've got to be willing to go with your gut, even amidst uncertainty, and it takes a confident and strong mindset to do that.

I have loved helping sick people get well, but today, although my work as a doctor is the same, my core underlying mission is much deeper than just healing sick people. People get sick and you take care of them. But now I want to make people healthy so that they don't get sick in the first place! It's a paradigm shift.

I consider it a huge privilege to be able to do what I do. When you're happy in your life's work, it does not feel like work. It is an absolute pleasure.

The only thing that keeps me from working all the time is my wife. I could do what I do 24/7 easily, but she keeps me grounded and helps me take time off for family and vacations. I love those things very much, but I'm also passionate about the work that I do.

As you read through these pages, I hope you'll recalibrate and start focusing on a healthier you by evaluating your mindset and lifestyle. Are the choices you've made lining up with the life you want to lead? Or are you in a hurry to retire and get off the "treadmill" of work? Retirement can be a double-edged sword. There are studies that show retirement is associated with decreased longevity.

Is it possible that people who are in a hurry to retire may not be working in their calling or doing what they are supposed to be doing? When you find what you're supposed to be doing in life, it feeds your soul.

Avoid the Myths

Since I've been educating individuals on their health and wellness, I've noticed the plethora of myths surrounding diet and exercise and even aging. There's just so many armchair physicians out there. There are people that will tell you that it would better for you to use artificial sweeteners rather than sugar. However, studies show that people who drink diet drinks in fact gain more weight than those who drink the same drink with sugar. The reason why is that it is believed that artificial sweeteners never shut down the brain's yearning for sugar, so you continue to crave more. Real sugar at least satisfies the brain at some point. But real sugar, especially in excessive amounts, is not good for you.

Aspartame, a common artificial sweetener in popular soft drinks, is a neurotoxin in high doses. Hello, dementia! Fat doesn't make you fat. Sugar makes you fat. So instead of compromising, how about deleting it all? Detox your diet and eliminate, eliminate, eliminate. You'll be amazed at how much better you feel when you do.

If you absolutely must choose to use an artificial sweetener, the best ones are stevia, xylitol, and erythritol. They are plant-based. The latter two are sugar alcohols and are minimally absorbed, if at all. They ferment in your gut by bacteria, which can cause gastrointestinal symptoms such as bloating, gas, and diarrhea. So, don't eat them too much.

There have been a lot of studies regarding stroke and vascular issues because of poor lifestyle decisions. The incidence of ischemic strokes in young people is rising, along with their cholesterol levels and high blood pressure. This is all lifestyle related.

Think about the daily choices you make and how they impact your health and family. How do you want your health to be now and in the future? How do you want your level of function to be now and in the future? A stroke is not my idea of healthy living.

The choice is always yours. You have to take control of your own health. You are responsible for it. If your doctor told you that you were at high risk for a cardiac episode, would you change your lifestyle to lower or eliminate the risk? Most people would answer yes. But believe it or not, it's simply not true. It's been my experience as a physician that patients often don't listen to the advice given, or initially they do, but eventually, they go back to their old ways. Therefore, if you're the one who adopts this knowledge about healthy living into your life and sticks to it, you'll be the exception and not the rule.

The American Association for Heart and Stroke did research that showed that 55 percent of patients at high risk were unwilling to change their poor lifestyle habits. Can you imagine having the power at your fingertips to make a positive change, maybe even having a wakeup call, and yet not implementing it?

It is all about lifestyle!

CHAPTER 6

THE AGING BRAIN

The human brain. What an amazing organ. I have been in love with the brain ever since I first I saw one while in surgery as a medical student at Johns Hopkins. It is who you are and where you live. It has the daunting task of taking in all of the sensory input provided to it by the outside environment through our various senses, creating the reality you see around you.

The brain is the most complex organ of the human body. It is responsible for everything that you do, from simple things like movement to complex abstract thinking. It is active 24/7, even when you're asleep. Contrary to what some people think, we use most of our brains most of the time, not just 10 percent. If you are using just 10 percent of your brain, then I feel sorry for you.

Ninety-five percent of brain activity is at the subconscious level, while 5 percent of cognition is at the conscious level. The average human brain weighs about 3 pounds and represents about 2 percent of the body weight, yet it uses 20 percent of the body's energy production. The brain has the consistency of firm jelly and is very fragile, so you have to be especially gentle when performing surgery on it. Your surgical technique must be meticulous, accurate, well planned, and perfectly precise. There is no room for error.

The brain contains about 86 billion brain cells (neurons). Each neuron has a cell body and a number of processes that project from the body in branch-like form called dendrites. The dendrites extend in all directions toward other brain cells where they communicate via electrical and chemical signals. Each neuron has an axon that projects from its body to make connections to many other neurons through which electrical signals travels. The neurons make up the gray matter of the brain, while the axons collectively make up the white matter of the brain.

The brain is the "fattiest" organ of the body. Sixty percent of the dry weight of the brain is made up of fat. The brain is made up of 75 percent water, while the human body is about 60–70 percent water. It takes only 2 percent brain dehydration to affect attention, memory, and cognition, so maintaining good hydration at all times is essential for healthy brain function.

The more you think, the more energy and oxygen the brain uses. So if you want to burn calories, keep thinking. The heart delivers 20–25 percent of your blood to your brain with each contraction, so keeping your blood vessels open and healthy is crucial to brain health.

The brain begins to age just like any other organ of the human body, but brain aging is not necessarily tied to chronologic aging. It is possible to slow biologic aging and reduce or prevent age-related chronic diseases, such as dementia. Taking steps to protect your brain from the ravages of aging should begin at an early age before irreversible changes occur. Once you lose it, it's hard to get it back. The brain begins to deteriorate surprisingly early in life. Gray matter volume begins to decrease after age twenty, possibly due to the death of neurons themselves or due to a decrease in their size and in the number of connections between them.

As we age, our brains get smaller. They begin to atrophy. The volume of the brain declines by 5 percent per decade after age 40. The rate of shrinkage may accelerate even more after age 70.

Shrinkage occurs in both the gray and white matter. White matter volume loss is greater than that of gray matter. In one autopsy study, subjects over 70 years showed a 16–20 percent decrease in white matter volume compared to younger subjects. Imagine one-fifth of your white matter gone by age 70.

The brain shrinks by different amounts in different areas. The frontal lobes, the area associated with judgment, shrink the most and are related to cognitive decline. The occipital lobes, which are related to vision, shrink the least. The hippocampus, which is located on the inside portion (medial) of the temporal lobe and is one of the areas of the brain associated with memory, also shrinks, affecting short-term memory. The frontal lobes are more affected in men, while the hippocampus and parietal lobes are more affected in women.

As the brain ages, cognitive decline can set in. The most common cognitive changes seen in brain aging is memory, especially recall (episodic memory) and semantic memory, the memory of what things mean. Other cognitive changes commonly seen include slower reaction times, decreased attention, and slower processing speeds.

A decrease in neurotransmitters is commonly observed with brain aging. Dopamine levels decline 10 percent per decade, beginning in early adulthood. Low levels of dopamine is associated with motor disorders such as Parkinson's disease as well as cognitive decline.

Brain function can be affected by declining hormone levels that commonly occur with normal aging, particularly the sex hormones. Women are especially affected. The incidence of Alzheimer's disease is greater in women than in men. Hormone replacement therapy both in men and women can be protective. Well-balanced and optimized hormones are good for the brain, so never take your hormones for granted.

Metabolic factors can affect brain aging. The aging brain has a decreased ability to metabolize sugar. Some have called this type 3 diabetes, where the brain has developed insulin resistance. This can cause accelerated brain aging with cognitive decline. Metabolic derangements are also responsible for increased free radical formation and oxidative stress, which lead to chronic brain inflammation and accelerated brain aging. The good thing is that there are steps you can take to reverse aging of the brain.

We've all heard a lot of frightening statistics. The incidence of stroke and dementia increase with increasing age. About 20 percent of 80 year olds have dementia, increasing to 40 percent by age 90. Alzheimer's disease accounts for 40–70 percent of dementias while vascular dementia accounts for 15–30 percent.

Alzheimer's disease is in part caused by metabolic problems at the cellular level, while vascular dementia is related to decreased blood flow to the brain, although there can be a lot of overlap given that poor lifestyle habits can affect both mechanisms.

The protein beta-amyloid is found to accumulate in the brain of all patients with Alzheimer's disease and is believed to cause the death of neurons. We find beta-amyloid accumulation in the brains of up to 20–30 percent of normal adults, which may place them at higher risk of developing cognitive impairment over time. We also find neurofibrillary tangles, which are aggregates of defective tau proteins and plaques in the brains of patients with Alzheimer's disease.

Alzheimer's and dementia are devastating diseases. Once diagnosed, they are gradually progressive. According to the Alzheimer's Association, 5.5 million Americans had Alzheimer's disease in 2017. Of these, 5.3 million were 65 or older. Ten percent of people 65 or older have Alzheimer's disease. Two-thirds of Alzheimer's patients are women. Total annual payments for healthcare in 2017 for all individuals with Alzheimer's disease was $259 billion. This is expected to increase to $1.1 trillion by 2050.

The risk of developing Alzheimer's disease doubles every five years starting at age 65. By age 85 years, 25–50 percent of people will show signs of the disease.

When it comes to dementia and Alzheimer's disease, an ounce of prevention is worth 10,000 pounds of cure. In fact, there is no cure. Once there is a diagnosis, there is limited treatment available at that point. As of this writing, there is no medication that can reverse or even stop the process. In general, patients progress over time to the point where they are bedridden and eventually die. It is heart-wrenching to watch the process both for the family and their healthcare givers. Prevention is the best approach. If we can eliminate the risk factors associated with dementia, we can reduce the prevalence of dementia in our population.

In a study presented at the 2017 Alzheimer's Association International Conference, Dr. Yian Gu found that people who consume more inflammatory food had smaller gray matter brain volume and had poorer scores on cognitive brain testing. They had higher levels of the inflammatory markers C-reactive protein and IL6 in their blood. There is a connection between diet and dementia as many foods modulate the inflammatory process.

You have a second brain in your gut, officially known as the enteric nervous system. It contains about 100 million neurons, more than the spinal cord. It communicates with your brain through the vagus nerve.

Diets consisting of fish, nuts, Omega 3 polyunsaturated fatty acids, and folate as well as Mediterranean-type diets were found in association with a lower risk for Alzheimer's disease. In a study by Tsivgoulis (*Neurology*, 2013 Apr 30), higher adherence to a Mediterranean diet lowered the likelihood of developing cognitive impairment in nondiabetics by 20 percent. The diet consisted of high consumption of vegetables, olive oil, nuts, and fish with a low intake of saturated fats, meat, and dairy.

Is the unhealthy food you are eating now really worth it? Do you really want to be an Alzheimer's statistic and have your brain shrink and your memories forgotten? The time to take action by adopting healthy lifestyle habits is now. Once you lose it, it is gone forever, so don't wait until it's too late.

According to a review of the world's literature by twenty-four experts for the Lancet Commission on Dementia Prevention, Intervention and Care presented in July 2017 at the Alzheimer's

Association International Conference in London, a dramatic 35 percent can reduce dementia risk by lifestyle modifications.

FORTY-SEVEN MILLION PEOPLE WORLDWIDE HAVE DEMENTIA. THIS NUMBER IS EXPECTED TO TRIPLE BY 2050.

Adopting healthy lifestyle habits can reduce your risk of dementia by over one-third. So what are you waiting for? Adopt those healthy habits now before your brain is permanently damaged.

Global cost of dementia in 2015 was $818 billion. Imagine what it will be in 2050. Potentially, it could be $2.4 trillion or more. If we can reduce the risk of dementia by 35 percent, that would have a profound effect on our population with millions of people maintaining normal cognitive function, interacting normally with friends and family, and living normal lives, rather than being residents of nursing homes requiring continuous care. Imagine how much of the 2.4 trillion dollars could be saved and put to better use somewhere else in the world economy?

Nine risk factors have been identified with dementia. Control these and you can lower your risk of dementia. The nine risk factors, as well as possible mechanisms, are presented in the table below:

Risk Factors: Possible Mechanisms

1. High blood pressure: vascular

2. Hearing loss: sensory deprivation

3. Obesity in middle age: inflammation

4. Smoking: inflammation, vascular

5. Physical inactivity: inflammation, vascular, lack of stimulation

6. Diabetes later in life: inflammation, vascular

7. Depression: possible hormonal imbalance, social isolation

8. Social isolation: sensory deprivation

9 Lower level of education: less brain and sensory stimulation

Your best protection from dementia is to adopt healthy lifestyle habits. Nothing else will work. No single drug will ever be able to reduce the risk of dementia by 35 percent. Only you can do that by adopting healthy lifestyle habits. If you don't make the changes now, you will be one of the statistics. How well do you want your brain to work as you get older? What level of function do you want to have? How do you want your friends and family to remember you?

Here are some immediate things you can do to prevent dementia:

1. Never stop learning. Stimulate your mind. The rewards are boundless. Learning new things will excite you and open up possibilities you never knew existed. An appetite for knowledge will keep your brain young.

2. Keep your blood vessels healthy so they can deliver oxygen and nutrients to your brain efficiently and remove cellular waste.

3. Stimulate all of your senses: sight, sound, touch, taste, and smell. Look at the beauty around you: nature, people, art, and music. We are surrounded by beauty. It's time to take notice. God created us and the world around us. These creations are beautiful. Take notice and enjoy them and be forever grateful for this gift.

4. Listen to the beauty around you. The sounds of people, nature, and music. What a joy! Image what it would be like without this.

5. Reach out and touch someone. It feels good. Touch is one of the oldest forms of communication.

6. Relish the taste of natural, wholesome foods including fruits, vegetables, and nuts. They contain the antioxidants and phytonutrients needed for optimal health.

7. Take in the smells of nature: flowers, forests, plants, oceans, and the wonderful smells after a rain.

8. We live in a beautiful world. Take in the gifts the world is giving you, and you will rejuvenate in mind, body, spirit, and soul.

9. Live a life of gratitude; it will bring you happiness. In my experience, happy people live longer with less cognitive decline.

10. Reduce chronic inflammation. Cognitive decline is directly related to chronic inflammation of not just the brain but the body as a whole. This is a major player in dementia and chronic diseases in general. Control inflammation, and you may live forever, including your brain.

11. Maintaining youthful hormonal balance is critical to good health, especially the health of your brain.

12. Keeping the body moving with exercise keeps the brain moving.

13. Don't smoke; this is an obvious one. If you are reading this book, then chances are you are not a smoker. Smoking is a sure way to get dementia and die. There are few things worse for your health than smoking. There is absolutely nothing good about smoking. It is all negative.

14. Control your blood pressure; be sure to have your doctor check your blood pressure on a regular basis. It is easy to treat in most cases. High blood pressure will cause

damage to your blood vessels, reducing blood flow to your brain, heart, and all organs of your body.

15. Get hearing aids as soon as possible if your hearing is impaired. Your brain needs all of the stimulation it can get, especially sound.

16. Control your weight. It will reduce inflammation, and you will be healthier for it. Remember, belly fat is especially inflammatory, so work on getting rid of that roll.

17. Develop and enjoy a great social life. Life is more fun when you share it with others, and your brain will love you for it.

18. Don't get diabetes. Diabetes will cause accelerated aging and increase your chances of getting dementia. Adopting healthy lifestyle habits will minimize this risk.

Prevention is the best approach. If we can eliminate the risk factors associated with dementia, we can reduce the prevalence of dementia in our population. Tackle one of these items at a time on the list or make the leap and do them all. Work right now to eliminate unhealthy habits from your life, and you'll see an immediate change in your energy levels and health!

CHAPTER 7

EXERCISE
AND AGING

Exercise, exercise, exercise!

Often when I say this to anyone over fifty, they will come up with a litany excuses. "But wait, doc, my knees hurt," or "I've got an injury that prevents me from exercising!" There's simply no excuse that should keep you from exercising. In fact, the less you do, the less you're going to do, and the unhealthier you're going to get. Don't stop moving. Don't stop exercising!

But it doesn't really matter what you do for your body if you continue to eat poorly. To put it bluntly, *you can't out-exercise a bad diet*! Having said that, I really want to encourage you to exercise, but you must eat right to get the results you are looking for. Exercise alone will not get you there.

It bears repeating: Good health doesn't happen by accident. It requires participation, which requires knowledge. Put your body first. It's the only one you have. Exercise regularly. What you don't use, you lose! Life isn't all about the number of years but the quality of them. We want to give you ten more healthy years—not ten years of inactivity and frailty!

We talked about centenarians earlier in the book to show you what's possible. You simply don't have to accept that you're only going to live seventy years. You're extraordinary, and you're reading this book. You can make massive, incredible changes today that will impact the rest of your days! What if I told you that it's possible for you to have the best sex life you've ever had in your sixth decade? I'm telling you that it's possible. Plenty of our patients have a renewed sexual life, enhanced energy, and a new outlook on life.

It's Not about How Long You Live

It's about the quality of the life you live. You want to be super productive and engaging. You don't want to sit and play cards. This requires a focus on health. I wanted to focus on my health because as a neurosurgeon, it's my performance that matters. I must be at the top of my game all the time. I cannot be average. You wouldn't want someone average working on your body! People may look at my lifestyle and exercise commitment of six days a week, even after a whole day of surgery, as extreme. But I bet if you had a child I was operating on, you wouldn't think taking care of my health was extreme.

As a neurosurgeon, you have to be at 100 percent, 100 percent of the time. If you have a 9-hour surgery, you can't get tired at the 6-hour mark because you still have 3 more hours to go, and often the difficult part of the operation is closer to the end rather than the beginning. Having the skill to do complex spinal surgery is my passion. Every patient is unique and different. No 2 cases are the same, so you need different solutions for different patients. I love being a problem solver, finding the solution, and executing with perfection to get a positive outcome. But it is a challenging specialty, and I've got to be able to function at this high level and fire on all cylinders, at all times!

You must practice healthy lifestyle habits to perform at the level required for what I do. Nutrition and exercise are so important for maintaining your edge. If I didn't take care of myself, I would not have the stamina and would not be able to do the difficult cases that I do. I didn't go to medical school, work hard, and study endlessly to give up now or make mistakes! In my line of work where I am often working under the operating microscope, decompressing a spinal cord while holding a drill that is spinning at 75,000 RPM, drilling off bone spurs that have grown into the spinal cord and moving the tip of the drill at submillimeter movements for six hours, you have to be on always. You have to be beyond 100 percent. You can't be worse at hour 6 than you were at hour 1. There are no cutting corners in neurosurgery. There is no room for error.

My job is to help people. There is no greater calling. I have been doing neurosurgery since 1980 and have no plans to stop. So, staying in top physical condition is very important for me so that I can continue to function at a high level.

I was saddened that Dr. Ben Carson, the renowned pediatric neurosurgeon from Johns Hopkins, retired at age sixty-two, even if it was to run for president. I had worked with Dr. Carson when I was a medical student at the Johns Hopkins University School of Medicine. He was a first-year resident, and I was his medical student. I had the good fortune to work closely with him. His skill, judgment, and knowledge base are now gone forever. You can't replace his experience. Judgement, surgical skills, and experience don't grow on trees. You can't replicate them or mass-produce them. They can only be acquired through time.

But the truth is, even if you're a taxi driver or a janitor, you still have to be focused on your health and living a healthy lifestyle because your health is the most valuable asset that you have. As a taxi or bus driver, you want to get your passengers to where they're going safely, instead of falling asleep at the wheel while driving.

If you're a janitor and you've got kids, how are you going to play with them at the end of the day if you've used up all your energy? No matter what kind of work you do, you cannot go wrong with a commitment to health. Think of how many things you miss out on when your energy is zapped and you are asleep on the couch.

Regardless of the form of exercise you choose, the physical and mental benefits are undeniable.

Physical Benefits of Exercise

As we age, the human body has a natural tendency to gain fat and lose bone mineral density, lean muscle, power, coordination, and balance. Regularly exercising slows and in many cases, reverses these physiologic changes of aging. Sarcopenia, osteoporosis, balance problems, and frailty are not inevitable and are preventable by committing to proper nutrition and a regular exercise program.

Strength training is any exercise that causes the muscles to contract against an external resistance with the expected outcome of increases in muscle tone, mass strength, or endurance. The form of resistance can range from body weight, resistance bands, free weights, or anything that causes the muscles to contract. Strength training causes small tears in the muscle cells, which are repaired during recovery. With muscles, testosterone, insulin-like growth factor (I-GF), growth hormone, protein, and other nutrients rush to the muscle after a resistance exercise session to help repair the muscles to make them stronger. Importantly, your muscles heal and grow when you aren't working out, and so that's why it's necessary to leave time between workouts for recovery. That is the reason that I alternate days between weight training and cardio. I also like to give each body region about one week to recover. For example, I do a chest workout on Mondays; back workout on Wednesdays; and arms and legs on Fridays. The in-between

> WHEN YOU LACK ENERGY, IT'S A DRILL TO GET UP EVERY DAY AND GO TO WORK. STAY PASSIONATE ABOUT LIFE. MAKE A COMMITMENT TO CHANGE AND ELIMINATE BAD HABITS TODAY.

days, I do cardio. The only exception is abs. I do those three times a week, the same days as weight training.

I graduated from medical school in 1979, and today I am still as excited about being a doctor, nearly four decades later, as I was then as a new medical graduate. As you might imagine, that in and of itself was a very exciting time! I have performed about 300 surgeries a year for the last 37 years. That equates to over 11,000 surgeries, and that number will continue to grow. I am not anywhere near retirement.

Surgeons should think carefully before retiring. Once you retire all that knowledge goes away. You spend so much time learning and training to be a neurosurgeon. The experience is irreplaceable. You have to live it to get it. There are no shortcuts. As such, it is priceless. Who your surgeon is, their experience, along with their skill level can make a huge difference in outcomes considering the complexity of neurosurgery and spine surgery in particular.

IT'S NOT ABOUT HOW LONG YOU LIVE IT'S ABOUT THE QUALITY OF YOUR LIFE.

Being a neurosurgeon for thirty-seven years, I have learned how important nutrition and exercise are before performing long, complex surgeries. Nutrition is important to maintain stable blood sugar levels throughout a case. A surgeon can't make good surgical decisions if he is hypoglycemic. You have to make sure that you are nutritionally sound. You can't have your blood sugar go up and down while you are performing surgery. It's not good for the surgeon or the patient.

Importance of Fitness as It Relates to Aging

The evidence is clear: exercise is the best anti-aging medicine there is. Regular exercise improves your physical and mental health, lowers your risk for chronic diseases such as diabetes and obesity, increases your lifespan, and naturally stimulates the release of hormones into your body. Individuals who participate in a regular exercise program feel stronger, younger, have more energy and libido, and overall are happier and more satisfied with their lives.

The table below shows some of the signs and symptoms of aging along with the positive effects exercise has on those symptoms (2).

Characteristic	Aging	Resistance Training
Muscular Strength	Decreases	Increases
Power	Decreases	Increases
Muscular Endurance	Decreases	Increases
Muscle Mass	Decreases	Increases
Muscle Fiber Size	Decreases	Increases
Muscular Metabolic Capacity	Decreases	Increases
Resting Metabolic Rate	Decreases	Increases
Body Fat	Increases	Decreases
Bone Mineral Density	Decreases	Increases
Physical Function	Decreases	Increases

Exercise Prescription

The American College of Sports Medicine (ACSM) calls regular exercise, beyond activities of daily living, essential for most adults. The ACSM's recommendations for exercise are considered the gold standard and are widely accepted among health and fitness professionals. Those recommendations are as follows (1):

- Thirty minutes of moderate-intensity cardiorespiratory exercise five days a week for a total of 150 minutes a week, vigorous-intensity cardiorespiratory exercise for 20 minutes a day, 3 days a week, or a combination of the 2.

- Two to three sessions a week of resistance exercises for each of the major muscle groups
- At least two days a week of flexibility

In summary, 150 minutes of cardiorespiratory exercise a week, 2 to 3 days of resistance exercise, and at least 2 days of flexibility exercises, such as yoga or stretching. Even if an individual cannot complete the full 150 minutes of cardio, any amount of exercise beyond the activities of daily living is considered beneficial. Exercise programs should always be modified to fit an individual's physical abilities, health status, functional abilities, and goals (5).

Terminology

Repetitions or Reps: One full movement of the exercise from start to the prescribed end-point and back to the original starting position.

Sets: This refers to the complete number of reps.

Positive phase: The positive phase is the part of the exercise that requires your muscles to contract. For example, when you are doing a bicep curl, the positive phase is when you flex your elbow and pull the weight up.

Negative phase: The negative phase of the exercise requires you to lower the weight to the starting position slowly. For example, when doing a bicep curl, the negative phase is when you extend your elbow and slowly lower back down until the arm is straight.

Lifting Speed

The speed a resistance exercise is performed plays a major role in the incidence of injury as well as in the strength and muscle development. Fast lifting creates momentum and often does not allow significant blood flow to the muscle. Slow movement through an exercise creates less momentum and less internal friction. I love lifting weights, but I'm moderate about it and don't overdo it. I lift weights for about sixty minutes a day, three days a week.

A good strength-training program requires an even powering of muscles throughout the range of motion that promotes blood flow to the specific muscle targets, with a bias toward slow rather than fast speed. A common mistake for beginning strength training is the tendency to lift weights too fast and in a jerky motion.

Each muscle has a positive phase where the muscle contracts and a negative phase where the muscle is returning to its original state. It is very important to make sure that the negative phase is two to three times longer than the positive phase. Generally, it is recommended that you spend one or two seconds for each positive lifting phase and three or four seconds for each negative lifting phase. If your motion is jerky or too fast, then you are not getting the maximum benefit from your program. Take your time and enjoy your workout. Find something you love to do and do it!

Frequency of Strength Training

A good general recommendation for the frequency of strength training is two to three times a week for thirty to forty-five minutes a session. Your objective also determines frequency; build muscle, endurance, or health improvement. A rest day should follow each day of strength training. Rest days are crucial to allow the muscles worked to rebuild and recover.

Benefits of Strength Training

There are numerous benefits to strength training. It can significantly reduce the symptoms of diseases and chronic conditions, such as:

- Arthritis
- Type II diabetes

- Osteoporosis
- Obesity
- Back pain
- Depression

With age, people begin to have trouble with balance and flexibility as well. When strength training exercises are done properly and through the full range of motion, they have been proven to improve flexibility and balance.

Strength Training and Longevity

Strength training is a crucial component to an anti-aging exercise program. Our body strength decreases by 6–10 percent each decade after age 30. By age 70 years, there is only about 50 percent of our body strength left. With a decrease in body strength, there is a decline in other areas as well, for example, less energy, less balance, and an accident rate increase. Strength training causes the pituitary gland to release growth hormone, which is an important anti-aging hormone, as well as the release of testosterone, both of which help to rebuild your lost muscle mass.

Increased Metabolic Rate

Individuals with a higher muscle mass have a higher metabolism. Adding muscle mass through strength training increases the basal metabolic rate. The basal metabolic rate is the number of calories your body utilizes at rest. Strength training can provide up to a 15 percent increase in metabolic rate. Incorporating a strength training routine allows you to burn a greater number of calories daily.

Improved Glucose Control

Over 14 million Americans have type II diabetes, a form of diabetes that is commonly associated with obesity but occurs even in normal weight people. Many more have insulin resistance also known as prediabetes. This is the precursor to type II diabetes. Diet and exercise can reverse and even prevent diabetes and prediabetes. Exercise can help enhance glucose metabolism. For instance, if we looked under the microscope at a muscle that has not been exercising and compared that muscle to one that has been exercising, we would see that there is an increase in the number of capillaries in the exercising muscle. With an increase in the capillary density, more blood flow to active muscle increases the efficiency of glucose metabolism. Typically, weight loss will improve the overall health of someone with type 2 diabetes and will decrease the need for insulin in those who are dependent on it.

Improved Sleep

Those who exercise regularly enjoy improved sleep quality. They fall asleep more quickly, awaken less often, and sleep more deeply and longer. When it comes to depression, the sleep benefits obtained because of strength training are comparable to treatment with medication.

Weight Loss/Control

A strength training regime is critical to a well-rounded exercise routine for weight loss. Cardio training alone will not provide an adequate boost to metabolism and calorie burn. Individuals with a higher muscle mass have a higher basal metabolic rate. Strength training allows your body to add more muscle that continues to burn off calories throughout the day. To burn more calories and boost metabolic rate, you have to develop more muscle mass. This is the metabolic engine that will burn calories and improve your body composition.

As you put on more muscle and lose fat, your body weight may not change, but your body composition will improve. Your percent of body fat will go down while your scale may remain the same. If you lose 10 pounds of fat and gain 10 pounds of muscle, your weight will stay the same, but your body composition will be greatly improved. The only way to tell is with a body composition scan. The body composition scan will tell you exactly how much fat you have lost and how much muscle mass (lean) you have gained down to the gram. It is through this mechanism that my percent body fat went from 21 percent to 6.7 percent while my weight stayed about the same. You have to measure along the way to see if you are getting the results that you are seeking. Without this measurement, it is like trying to navigate without a compass or nowadays GPS.

Increased Bone Mineral Density

Strength training over a period of time will prevent not only the loss of bone mineral density but also will work to rebuild bone matter. Bone mineral density hits its peak at age thirty and then begins to decline after that. This can be delayed or even prevented if weight-bearing exercises like those used in a strength training program are initiated. The loading of bone signals the bone cells to store more calcium so as to build more bone and make it stronger.

Reduced Risk of Injury

The nice thing about strength training is that it strengthens everything, not just your muscles and bones. When you lift weights, you also strengthen connective tissue—the ligaments and tendons that hold your bones together and keep your body moving well on a regular basis. Strengthening your connective tissue will help you continue to operate in peak condition and protect your body from injuries.

With age, the structures of the heart can become weaker, more rigid, and less resilient. The heart fills and empties more slowly, putting less blood volume into circulation with each contraction. The arteries and arterioles in our heart that are responsible for delivering blood and oxygen to heart cells become thicker and less elastic. These factors, combined with the increase in arterial plaque buildup that comes with an unhealthy diet, cause the heart to become much more susceptible to heart disease and blockages that can cause a heart attack and in the brain, a stroke.

During exercise, the body experiences an increased heart rate, oxygen uptake, systolic blood pressure, blood flow to active muscles, and stroke volume (amount of blood your heart pumps out). In the long term, exercise can decrease your heart rate at rest and during submaximal exercise. Your heart is a muscle. When you exercise your body, you are also exercising your heart muscle. It becomes stronger and more efficient and can pump more blood with each contraction. It, therefore, doesn't need to contract as often to get the same amount of blood circulating throughout your body, so it contracts less often per minute. As a result, your resting pulse goes down when you exercise regularly. It is a sign that you are in better health and making progress.

With a lower pulse, your heart will not have to work as hard to pump blood to your muscles and organs. This reduced stress on your heart lowers your risk for a multitude of cardiovascular events. Individuals who exercise regularly also develop an increase in left ventricular wall thickness and mass. The heart muscle actually enlarges with exercise just like your biceps or triceps. As it is stronger, it can pump more blood per contraction and contract less frequently. Exercise improves the resilience of your heart as you age.

Cardiovascular Training

Cardiovascular training (aerobic exercise) is a critical component of the age-management program. There are many benefits: increase in muscle mass and strength, loss of fat, increase in energy, and a decrease in anxiety and depression. Cardiovascular training also increases the good cholesterol (HDL), lowers blood pressure, and most importantly, improves the immune system. These benefits protect the body from cardiovascular diseases, hypertension, stroke, diabetes, and osteoporosis.

A study at Harvard University found that as the physical activity of men increased, their death rate decreased. Those who engaged in moderate exercise, at least 2000 calories per week, decreased their overall death rate by 25–33 percent and decreased their risk of coronary artery disease by 41 percent! Moderate level exercise such as jogging, swimming, and tennis is the key to longevity. While selecting an aerobic exercise program, we consider the type of activity, the duration of activity, the frequency of activity, the intensity of activity, and the progression.

Duration and Frequency

It is recommended that you aim to burn 2000 calories each week. If you are performing weight training 40 to 60 minutes 3 times a week, you will burn close to 750–900 calories total. This will leave you with 1100–1250 calories to expend during aerobic exercise. We recommend you perform resistance training 3 times a week and cardiovascular training 3 times a week. This allows the body to recover, providing protection from oxidative stress and tissue damage, which causes muscle wasting and aging.

Maximum Heart Rate

At birth, maximum heart rate is equal to 220 beats per minute. Every year, maximum heart rate decreases by one beat per minute. The maximum targeted heart rate is simply 220 minus your age. A person, age 2, has a maximum heart rate of 218. A person, age 20, has a maximum heart rate of 200. A person age 50 has a maximum heart rate of 170, and so forth. It is recommended that you do not exceed your maximum heart rate.

During cardiovascular training, your goal should be to partially stress your heart but not to overstress it. Each cardiovascular workout should include a warmup and cooldown period at 60 percent of your maximum heart rate. The time spent training close to your maximum should be minimal at the start of your program. As the heart becomes stronger, your ability to train for longer periods closer to your maximum heart rate will improve over time. The cardiovascular program is designed to slowly increase your time spent at or near your maximum heart rate.

Intensity

Intensity is expressed as a percentage in terms of your maximum heart rate. It is recommended that you exercise within a range of 60–95 percent of your maximum heart rate. If you are 60 years old, then your maximum heart rate is 160 (220–60). Therefore, if you are training at 60–95 percent of your maximum heart rate, then 60 percent of 160 equals 96 (160 x 0.60), and 95 percent of 160 equals 152 (160 x 0.95). Your target heart rate range will be 96–152. Most cardiovascular machines are equipped with heart rate monitors.

Personal heart rate monitors, however, are more accurate, and you can customize them to your needs. I recommend that you always monitor your heart rate while doing cardio so that you know what your heart rate is at all times so as to keep it in the recommended range. Without measuring it, you won't know.

Cardiovascular Zones

The goal when training in zones is to keep your heart in a healthy condition and challenge yourself. In Zone 1 and 2, you are increasing endurance and functional capacity. There will be an increase in the number and size of blood vessels in these zones. In Zone 3, the intensity is high and more calories are burned per minute. Short bursts in Zone 3 and Zone 4 are ideal, but prolonged periods in these zones are not recommended. Interval training is permitted as small bursts to challenge the heart. However, overtraining in Zone 3 and 4 can overstress the heart. In Zone 4, the highest numbers of calories are burned per minute, but as stated before, it is unrealistic and unhealthy to train in this zone for prolonged periods. It is generally recommended that if you are just starting to exercise from a sedentary lifestyle that you increase intensity 5–10 percent each month. The majority of a beginner's time should be spent in Zone 1, with small bursts into higher zones being permitted.

Zone 1: 60–70 percent of maximum heart rate
85 percent calories burned are fat
10 percent calories burned are carbohydrates
5 percent calories burned are protein

Zone 2: 70–80 percent of maximum heart rate
50 percent calories burned are from fat
50 percent calories burned are from carbohydrates
<1 percent calories burned are from protein

Zone 3: 80–90 percent of maximum heart rate
85 percent calories burned are from carbohydrates
15 percent calories burned are from fat
<1 percent calories burned are from protein

Zone 4: 90–100 percent of maximum heart rate
90 percent calories burned are from carbohydrates
10 percent calories burned are from fat
<1 percent calories burned are from protein

Aerobic Workout

Warmup Phase

This phase includes light movement and stretching. Light movement includes low intensity (50–60 percent) walking, low-intensity cycling, or low-intensity elliptical training. This phase usually lasts about 5 minutes. The purpose of the warmup phase is to slowly increase the body temperature, loosen the joints, and loosen tight muscles. Failure to provide the body with a proper warmup will lead to injury. Stretch.

Workout Phase

This phase can last anywhere from twenty-five to fifty minutes. Aerobic exercise of low to moderate intensity with small bursts is recommended to improve cardiovascular fitness and increase weight loss. Because exercise increases metabolism and therefore increases the production of free radicals and oxidative stress, which can cause aging, it is recommended that you consume plenty of antioxidants, which helps combat this damage, an unavoidable byproduct of exercise.

> REGARDLESS OF THE EXERCISE YOU CHOOSE, DO SOMETHING. DON'T MAKE IT COMPLEX. FIND WHAT YOU LOVE AND DO IT.

Cooldown Phase

This phase, like the warmup phase, usually lasts five minutes and consists of low-intensity exercise. This allows the body to return to its normal resting level. The cooldown period allows the heart to adjust to the decreased demand for blood flow and oxygen. It is also a good time to stretch.

Interval Training

Interval training consists of repeated intervals of low-medium intensity, 60–80 percent of maximum heart rate, flanked by short bursts of high-intensity sprints at 80–100 percent maximum heart rate. This type of training is beneficial because it trains the body to adapt to different stressors. Interval training also increases the basal metabolic rate (BMR) postexercise for up to 48 hours. It is especially good if you want to reduce body fat as you continue to burn fat even after you exercise up to 48 hours later.

While cardiovascular training provides an important part to your overall wellness, it must be combined with resistance training, proper supplementation, and a low glycemic nutrition program.

Measuring Progress

The scale is not a good indicator of your fat loss because it does not show the exchange of fat for muscle. Muscle is denser than fat and therefore weighs more. The accurate measurement of lean muscle mass and fat mass, as well as percent body fat, is best determined by a Lunar iDXA body composition scan.

The Lunar iDXA Total Body Scan

- Provides comprehensive analysis of fat, muscle, and bone mass
- Determines regional body fat distribution
- Determines areas of strength and weakness allowing for more specific workouts
- Determines bone density in the fight against Osteoporosis
- Is an 8-minute total body scan—safe, comfortable, and painless
- Results are immediately available in real time

The Lunar iDXA body scan offers insight that traditional methods cannot. It accurately measures body fat and lean muscle mass to precisely determine your body fat percentage by region of your body. This allows me to create specific exercise and nutrition goals for my patients. The iDXA body scan looks beyond traditional BMI to determine body fat distribution.

> AN EXERCISE PROGRAM IS YOUR MOST IMPORTANT MEDICINE. START ONE TODAY.

With quarterly body composition measurements, we are able to tell if we are heading in the right direction and getting the results that we are looking for. It gives us an early warning sign if we are going in the wrong direction.

Musculoskeletal Health

Tendons and ligaments in the body become stiffer and lose their flexibility as we age. A sedentary lifestyle leads to a loss in muscle mass and, as a result, a decrease in strength, power, and resting metabolic rate. Bone mineral density decreases, increasing the chance of a bone fracture. Flexibility also decreases, increasing the risk for injury.

The body responds directly to the stress placed upon it via the concept of specificity. The muscles and joints stressed during exercise are the ones that in turn adapt and become stronger. As you age, your body loses the ability to produce strength and power through the loss of lean muscle mass (a condition called sarcopenia). Resistance training causes an increase in lean muscle mass and an increase in tensile strength in tendons and ligaments. These changes increase your ability to produce strength and power, allowing you to complete everyday tasks, like walking to the mailbox or picking up a box, with ease.

Weight-bearing activities such as walking, running, and playing sports increase the bone mineral density (BMD) that is slowly lost as we age, especially in women. When the bone density reaches a dangerously low level, it is classified as a disease known as osteoporosis that can cause spontaneous fractures of your bones, especially your hips and spine vertebra. In response to the mechanical stress placed on bones during exercise, the bone increases in mass and strength in order to support the stress being placed on it, thus improving BMD. Alternatively, inactivity or a sedentary lifestyle decreases bone mineral density and increases the chance of an injury. Activities such as running or walking are excellent for stimulating an increase in bone mineral density in the femur, knees, and bones of the lower leg. Studies have shown that in order to avoid low bone mineral density in old age, individuals should exercise in early adulthood to maximally elevate their peak bone mass. The denser your bones are, the stronger they will be going into old age.

A regular stretching program is important to maintain flexibility and decrease the chances of injury, especially while doing everyday tasks. For example, at a young age, quick reaction time and strength allows you to catch something that gets knocked off the counter. As you age and become less limber, lunging to catch something that falls off a table can result in a muscle tear or potentially even a fall.

Exercising improves your body composition, increasing muscle mass and reducing total body fat and especially intra-abdominal fat, which is associated with a higher risk for chronic diseases such as cardiovascular disease, high cholesterol, type II diabetes, and obesity. Individuals who exercise regularly also develop improvements in coordination, balance, and reaction time, all of which decline with age.

Mental Benefits of Exercise

Extensive testing has been done to evaluate the effect of exercise as a nonpharmacological treatment option for chronic diseases and conditions such as insomnia, anxiety, and depression.

Study after study shows that exercise reduces the symptoms of depression. One study examined thirty clinically depressed men and women. Members of the group were randomly assigned to an exercise group, a social support group, and a control group. Individuals in the exercise group completed twenty to forty minutes of walking just three times a week for six weeks. Results showed that the exercise program alleviated overall symptoms of depression and was more effective than the other two groups at reducing the symptoms. A separate twelve-month exercise versus control group study showed that the positive effects of exercise had continued at a follow-up twelve months later. Exercising improves not only mental health but also increases feelings of well-being and life satisfaction as you age.

Exercise releases endorphins, which are the chemicals in your brain that act as natural painkillers, your body's natural morphine. They are responsible for the "natural high" that is known to come with exercise. As we age and life becomes stressful, levels of the stress hormone cortisol become higher in the blood. High levels of cortisol can lead to a depressed immune system, high blood sugar, low libido, hypertension, and other undesirable symptoms. Exercise naturally reduces cortisol levels, lowering levels of stress and anxiety without the use of medication.

Of perhaps the utmost importance is the effect exercise has on sleep. As you age, it becomes harder to fall asleep and stay asleep. You may try different mattresses and special pillows and still not be able to find relief. Studies show that individuals who exercise regularly experience higher quality, more satisfying sleep. In individuals with sleep apnea, exercise reduces the severity of sleep apnea as well as improves cardiorespiratory fitness, decreases daytime sleepiness, and increases sleep efficiency. (6)

The figure below depicts the prevalence of insufficient rest or sleep for more than fourteen days of the last thirty days among US adults. (3)

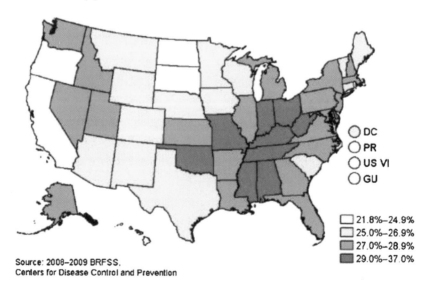

Source: 2008–2009 BRFSS,
Centers for Disease Control and Prevention

When compared to the below map of the prevalence of obesity in the United States, the connection is clear (7).

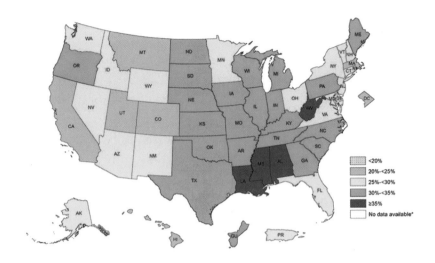

Sedentary, overweight individuals experience a lower quality of sleep and higher incidence of mental health issues when compared to their active counterparts. Maintaining your fitness as you age improves your sleep quality, reduces feelings of anxiety and stress, and overall improves your quality of life.

Effect of Exercise on Hormones

As we age, changes in the body's endocrine system occur naturally. The endocrine system works to establish homeostasis, or balance, in the human body through hormones. As you get older, levels of many hormones decline, some to critical levels. Your organs also become less sensitive to the hormones that are circulating in the body. With age, testosterone levels in both men and women decrease. In women progesterone and estradiol begin to decrease as they reach perimenopause and menopause. These hormones play a multitude of roles in the body, including maintenance of the internal environment, growth and development, libido, energy production, utilization and storage of fat, as well as maintaining muscle mass and bone density. (2)

During aerobic and resistance training, the body's internal balance is disrupted. In response, the endocrine system releases hormones to adapt and restore the balance to physiological functions. These adaptations include how much of a hormone is made, how much is stored, and the transportation and dissemination of the hormones throughout the body. It also determines the number of hormone receptors present on cell membranes where hormones attach. The primary hormones affected by exercise are testosterone and growth hormone. Exercise, especially vigorous exercise, is a great way of raising the levels of both.

Testosterone

Production of testosterone naturally slows as you age. It usually begins at age 30, and it's downhill from there. Testosterone in men typically declines by 1–3 percent per year, starting at age 30. These lower levels of testosterone are associated with depression, lower libido, irritability, fatigue, sexual dysfunction, brain fog, osteoporosis, and other undesirable effects, including insulin resistance. Exercise naturally stimulates the release of testosterone to initiate protein synthesis and muscle building. The development of lean muscle mass increases your resting metabolic rate, allowing you to burn more calories at rest. It also maintains your levels of strength and power and helps prevent injury as you age. Even a few heavy resistance exercise sessions can increase the number of testosterone receptors present in the muscle, making your body more sensitive to the testosterone available in the blood. For men who do resistance training regularly, studies support an overall sustained increase in resting serum testosterone concentrations. (2)

Growth Hormone

Growth hormone (GH) is another hormone whose release is stimulated by resistance training. Some of the physiological roles of GH include glycogen synthesis with decreased glucose utilization, increased protein synthesis, increased utilization of fatty acids, increased fat breakdown, increased collagen synthesis, and more. In layman's terms, GH helps build muscle, burn fat, and increase collagen made in the body, which helps give your skin strength and elasticity. Growth hormone is plentiful in children and young adults, but production tapers off as we age.

The hormones epinephrine, norepinephrine, and dopamine are also stimulated as a response to exercise. These hormones increase force production, increase muscle contraction rate, increase blood pressure and blood flow, and increase energy availability. (2) Maintaining your fitness as you age will allow you to feel younger and healthier, perform better, and have more energy than your sedentary age-matched counterpart. Try it; it works!

The physical, mental, and hormonal benefits improve your quality of life as well as health span and ultimately your lifespan. When it comes to aging, an exercise program is your most important medicine.

CHAPTER 8

HORMONES
AND AGING

Without hormones, mankind would be extinct. There would be no libido and no interest in reproducing. Hormones are perhaps the most overlooked and misunderstood aspect of longevity and aging well. It is not uncommon for people to come see me with a variety of ailments, many of which are related to hormone imbalances. Understanding how hormones work in your body is important. Hormones—well-balanced hormones—are essential for healthy aging. There are good hormones and bad hormones. Optimizing both to healthy levels is critical to health, longevity, and aging.

In the 1800s people often didn't live past 50 years of age, so endocrine issues were rarely a problem. Around age 50 is when you start to notice the effects of a declining endocrine system. Your endocrine system is a collection of endocrine glands that secrete hormones directly into your bloodstream. When we start feeling old, it is partly because of declining hormone levels. People didn't know about this decline in the 1800s because they didn't live long enough to feel the effects of lower hormone levels. They did not have the tools and technology that we have today to measure hormone levels with a simple, easy blood test.

Modern medicine has made it possible for us to live longer but, in many cases, not better. The idea is to create optimal health for your entire life, not just the first half.

Today we've seen advances in medicine that allow us to measure, track, and monitor hormones. When our hormone levels drop, we now have the means to restore them back to healthy, youthful levels. Why settle for a lower level of function with suboptimal hormone levels? We can change the way we feel and function by maintaining our hormones at optimal youthful levels but still well within the normal range. Why not be at your best? Why feel and look old if you don't have to? There is a better way to age. After treating well over 2000 patients in my age-management/anti-aging program, I have seen firsthand the transformations in health and wellness that can be achieved by restoring hormones to their youthful, optimal levels along with diet, exercise modifications, and nutritional supplements. After all, when did you feel and function at your best? When you were 25 or 30 years of age, or now when you are 50 or 60 years of age? By participating in a well-thought-out age-management program, we can make up for what we have lost.

Just because you are aging, that doesn't mean you have to feel old. Those who accept that are missing a lot. It doesn't have to be that way. There are ways to maintain a youthful body and mind despite physical age. When your hormones are at optimal levels, your productivity improves and in many cases can go through the roof. Many of my patients have reported much better energy, clearer thinking, improved libido, better mental focus, and a youthful outlook on life. Imagine adding these benefits to the wisdom you have acquired through life experiences. That is a powerful combination from which you can really accomplish a lot. When we are young, we have hormones but less wisdom. When we get older, we have wisdom but fewer hormones. Wouldn't it be great to have both? Well, now there is a way.

As a society, we have figured out how to live longer but not better. It's my quest to change all of that and deliver better healthcare. We should not have to feel old to be old. We can be old and feel good. One of the common myths I hear from people, in general, is that they feel as if their own lack of energy is due to the normal aging process and is inevitable. They settle for a lower level of function, thinking there is no way to get it back. Why settle for frailty and feebleness? There is a better way.

With lifestyle modifications, including correct diet, exercise, nutritional supplementation, and hormone optimization, you can lift that listless feeling, brain fog, and lack of get-up-and-go. You can even combat depression. It is about finding the root cause of your health issues versus treating the symptoms. It is impossible to be your best and function at optimal levels if your hormones are not where they should be. It is a huge key to success in the age-management process. You are only as old as your hormones. If your hormones are at youthful levels, you feel young. If they are at aged levels, you feel old. How do you want to feel?

The optimal level of a particular hormone depends on the hormone. Some hormones are optimal when they are in the upper range of normal, and some hormones are optimal when they are in the lower range of normal.

Insulin is one hormone we want at the lower range. Insulin is produced in the islet cells of the pancreas. It is involved in regulating blood sugar. In the presence of insulin, it is impossible to burn fat. Insulin promotes fat storage. It is responsible for controlling elevated blood sugar (glucose). In the presence of insulin, whatever sugar that is present in the blood that cannot be metabolized for energy is first converted to glycogen and stored in your muscle and liver. Once glycogen stores are filled up, sugar is converted to triglycerides and stored as fat. The longer insulin hangs around, the more your fat cells grow and the bigger your stomach gets. Insulin is also inflammatory partly because it increases fat stores. Fat promotes chronic inflammation.

The way to control insulin is through what we eat. It is our diet that will determine our insulin levels. Sugar in our diet, in all its forms, causes a dramatic rise in insulin. The less sugar in our diet, the lower our insulin levels are, and the better we can burn fat for fuel. That is why a low glycemic diet works so well to reduce body fat. By eating sugar, we are constantly feeding our fat stores. Fat doesn't make you fat; sugar makes you fat (by way of insulin)!

Whenever I introduce a new food to my diet and I am not sure if it will raise my blood sugar or not, I usually will check it with a glucometer, a device that measures blood sugar with a finger stick. It gives instantaneous results. Glucometers are commonly used by diabetic patients to check their blood sugar. It gives me valuable information as to how different foods affect my blood sugar.

Cortisol is another hormone that we typically like to see in the lower to mid-range of normal. Cortisol is produced in the adrenal glands located just above the kidneys. Cortisol is a stress hormone. It rises and falls with stress. With acute stress, it rises, and when the stress is gone, it declines back to normal. With chronic stress, it can remain elevated for longer periods of time, sometimes indefinitely. Chronically elevated cortisol is bad for your health.

It can suppress your immune system, making you more susceptible to infection and even cancer. It raises your blood sugar, and as a result, also raises your insulin levels, which in turn cause fat accumulation. It makes your skin thin and fragile, friable, and prone to bruising. It can even cause osteopenia and osteoporosis. It also zaps you of your energy. In extreme cases, you can develop adrenal fatigue where your adrenal glands are so overworked that they give up and stop producing enough cortisol. This can lead to extreme fatigue. In this situation, cortisol replacement may be necessary.

The way to lower elevated cortisol levels is by eliminating the stress if possible. Stress causes activation of the sympathetic nervous system. The sympathetic nervous system is responsible for our fight-or-flight response through the action of adrenaline and noradrenaline. Meditation is often very helpful in treating stress. It activates the parasympathetic nervous system through the vagus nerve. This counteracts and opposes the sympathetic nervous system and thus has a calming effect.

When it comes to your sex hormones, especially testosterone, we like to see it in the top quartile of the normal range. In my experience, men function much better when their testosterone levels are in that range, rather than the lower quartile. Your hormones are at their highest levels when you are in your twenties. When you hit 30, they begin to decline. Testosterone begins to decline 1–3 percent per year once you hit 30. By the time you are 50 years of age, your testosterone level may be down by 60 percent. As mentioned earlier, low testosterone can bring on a multitude of health problems, including insulin resistance, fat accumulation around the belly, diminished libido, diminished sexual function, loss of muscle mass, loss of energy, brain fog, loss of initiative, and diminished mood, as well as osteoporosis to name a few.

IF YOU WANT MORE SEX, MORE ENERGY, OR MORE VITALITY, START EXERCISING MORE. YOUR LIBIDO AND DESIRE WILL INCREASE AND SO WILL YOUR PERFORMANCE. NOW GO TAKE THAT WALK AROUND THE BLOCK OR JOG ON THE TREADMILL!

The expression "grumpy old men" comes from the fact that low testosterone can affect men's moods and make them irritable and grumpy. Restoring testosterone to normal youthful levels is a mood stabilizer for most men. Men with normal testosterone levels are generally happy people. They are happy because they function well and feel good. Who wouldn't be happy under the same circumstances? It comes down to the question: "Where would you like your hormone levels to be"? I know where I want mine.

Restoring testosterone to optimal levels will alleviate many of the medical issues noted. It will help restore lost muscle mass, improve bone density, improve libido and sexual function, improve mood, and improve sugar metabolism by muscle cells, thus improving insulin resistance and belly fat accumulation. Energy and brain fog are usually dramatically better as well. I have never seen a case of "steroid rage" in anyone. One patient (out of over 1000) reported slight irritability that resolved with lowering his dose slightly. In my experience, testosterone replacement therapy has been safe and effective without increased risk of heart attack, stroke, prostate cancer, or blood clots. It has dramatically improved the quality of life of my patients.

There are a lot of myths floating around out there about hormones and their impact on your body. At times, I encounter people who think that testosterone is bad for you. It is actually the opposite. Low testosterone levels are bad for you. Normal optimal testosterone levels are good for you.

Some falsely believe that testosterone replacement therapy in men will give them prostate cancer. This simply is not true. In medical studies, the incidence of prostate cancer was higher in the group of men within the lower quartile of the normal range as opposed to the group of men in the upper quartile. Translated another way, what these studies showed was that men with higher testosterone levels tended to get less prostate cancer than men with lower testosterone levels. Looking at this another way, testosterone may actually be protective of prostate cancer as men with higher levels tend to get prostate cancer less often than those with lower levels. Where do you want your testosterone level to be?

There have been isolated reports that testosterone may cause an increase in heart attacks. The vast majority of the medical literature simply does not bear this out. There are literally hundreds if not thousands of articles that show just the opposite: testosterone is beneficial for your heart and with good reason. Your heart is a muscle. Testosterone is good for muscles.

Testosterone is also good for your brain. The two parts of your body that have the most concentration of testosterone receptors are your heart and your brain. There must be a good reason for that; God doesn't make mistakes. Testosterone is important not only for your muscle but for your brain and heart as well. In fact, all the organs of the body have testosterone receptors. Maintaining healthy levels of testosterone is important for your body to function well. Testosterone protects you from insulin resistance. It enables muscles to metabolize sugar better.

I have seen restoring testosterone to optimal levels bring people back to life in the setting of a well-thought-out age-management program. Replacing hormones by themselves in a vacuum doesn't work nearly as well. It takes lifestyle modification including diet, exercise, and nutritional supplementation in addition to hormone balancing and optimization to get the most dramatic results.

The best way to measure testosterone is to measure how much testosterone is actually inside of a cell, which is where testosterone does its job. Unfortunately, we have no way to measure that, so we have to use the next best things: blood tests and our clinical judgment. We have to see how our patient is doing clinically and correlate that to the blood tests and the lifestyle modifications put in place. Are we getting the results that we are looking for? If not, why not? It's a doctor-patient partnership. In the end, it's the clinical response that matters the most.

To gain muscle mass, it takes much more than having adequate testosterone levels. Testosterone by itself won't do much. Testosterone acts as a catalyst. It makes it possible for you to gain muscle mass, but it won't happen unless you actually use that muscle through exercise and feed that muscle with proper nutrition. You have to eat plenty of protein as protein contains amino acids, the building blocks of muscle tissue. You also have to do weight training and use your muscles.

Without resistance training, your muscle mass will not increase. If I gave you testosterone and all you did was sit in a chair, nothing would happen. You would not increase your muscle mass or lose fat. You have to do it all to get the effect you are looking for. You must take control of your own health. Only you can do that. What do you want your body composition to be? Lifestyle and diet are very important aspects of maintaining your hormones and your health.

EXERCISE RELEASES ENDORPHINS, WHICH ARE THE CHEMICALS IN YOUR BRAIN THAT ACT AS NATURAL PAINKILLERS, YOUR BODY'S NATURAL MORPHINE. THEY ARE RESPONSIBLE FOR THE "NATURAL HIGH" THAT IS KNOWN TO COME WITH EXERCISE. AS WE AGE AND LIFE BECOMES STRESSFUL, LEVELS OF THE STRESS HORMONE CORTISOL BECOME HIGHER IN THE BLOOD.

While low testosterone can cause erectile dysfunction (ED), so can vascular disease. Vascular disease commonly presents with ED. Exercise also impacts your mental health and the way you feel about intimacy.

There is a strong correlation between sexual function and the health of your blood vessels. Good sexual health usually correlates with good cardiovascular health. Erectile dysfunction can be the first sign of cardiovascular disease. It's all about blood flow, especially when the penis is involved. Every organ needs blood flow to do its job properly: your brain, your heart, and your penis. Hence the saying good health, good sexual function! Poor lifestyle choices clog your arteries while healthy lifestyle choices open them up. What do you want your blood vessels to look like—soft, pliable and widely open allowing lots of blood to flow through them, or hard as a rock and partially closed off with reduced blood flow to your tissues?

In women, sex hormone replacement therapy usually involves bioidentical estrogen and progesterone in addition to bioidentical testosterone. *Bioidentical* means that they have the same chemical structure as the hormones your body makes. There has been concern that hormone replacement therapy in women increases the risk of breast cancer. This is only true for synthetic hormones, some of which contain horse estrogen and artificial progesterone known as progestin. This is not true for bioidentical estrogen and progesterone. The scientific literature shows that bioidentical estradiol and progesterone do not increase the risk of breast cancer. Synthetic estrogen and progestins (progestins are synthetic progesterone) are the hormones that have been associated with an increased breast cancer risk. Estrogen used by itself without progesterone may also increase the risk of breast cancer. The reason is that estrogen promotes the growth of tissue while progesterone promotes the development of that tissue, thus controlling its growth. Uncontrolled growth can be dangerous.

Despite what many doctors believe, even in women who have had hysterectomies, estradiol should not be used without also using progesterone. In men, progesterone may be protective for prostate cancer as it promotes development over growth. It is uncontrolled growth that causes cancer. To be at your best, your hormones have to be at their best, and that means you've got to understand and monitor your levels regularly.

Optimal hormone levels are different for each person, and that's an important factor to note when you're embarking on an age-management program. What may be optimal for one may not be for another. Different patients have different responses. An optimal level is that level where *you* feel and function at your best. The numbers are a starting point, but you really have to pay attention to the clinical response; that is the most important.

As a doctor, you can't always go by the numbers. What really matters is how the patient is doing. That is why hormone therapy should be a custom program unique for each and every patient.

Hormone list:

- Insulin
- Total testosterone
- Free testosterone
- Bioavailable testosterone
- Sex hormone-binding globulin (the hormone that binds testosterone)
- Luteinizing hormone
- Estradiol
- Cortisol (stress hormone)
- IGF-1 (proxy for growth hormone)
- PSA (in men to follow their prostate health)
- DHEA
- Follicle stimulating hormone
- Progesterone
- Estradiol
- Thyroid hormones (stress impacts your thyroid): TSH (thyroid stimulating hormone), Free T3, Free T4

The reason we measure for three values for testosterone is that total testosterone includes total and free testosterone. When testosterone is bound to protein, it can't bind with a cell receptor and thus cannot do its job. It is the free testosterone, the bioavailable testosterone, that is able to attach to the testosterone receptor on the cell membrane and do its job.

Testosterone that is bound to protein has no biological activity as the protein that is binding it is not letting it do its job. We also measure sex hormone binding globulin (SHBG). This is the protein that binds testosterone and keeps it from being active. If you have high levels of SHBG, it could mean that you don't have enough free testosterone to bind with the cell receptors even if your total testosterone level is normal. That is why it is important to measure both total and free testosterone. Free testosterone is the more important of the two. You may have to push total testosterone to higher levels to get adequate levels of free testosterone for your body to use. This is what is doing all of the work.

Hormones are like an orchestra. They work in unison to produce a symphony. You can't just look at one. You have to look at all of them because they work together. When you aren't producing enough of something, you will see differences in how your body functions. My role is to be the conductor and help the body maintain optimal function by monitoring your progress and making changes where needed.

In some men, as they get older, an interesting thing can happen: their testosterone levels drop while their estrogen levels go up. I sometimes see couples where the husband's estrogen level is higher than his wife's. She's in menopause and has lost her estrogen. He's accumulated belly fat and, as a result, has raised his estrogen levels. It's not uncommon for the men to develop gynecomastia (man boobs) once their estradiol levels go up. This is readily treatable through a comprehensive age-management program. Through lifestyle modifications and hormone balancing, this can all be reversed.

I can usually tell a lot about a patient's lifestyle by looking at their blood work. Blood work can tell us a lot about what is happening in their life. When we see their cortisol levels go up (stress hormone) and their thyroid levels drop (thyroid hormone is responsible for your metabolism), we know that stress is probably impacting their life. Stress not only raises your cortisol levels, but it also reduces thyroid function. This combination can really drain your energy.

When a woman enters menopause, her estrogen and testosterone levels drop. Estrogen protects women from cardiovascular disease. After menopause, that protection is lost. The leading cause of death in women after menopause isn't breast cancer or any other cancer; it is cardiovascular disease. Artificial progestins (synthetic hormones) are what can increase their risk for breast cancer.

Women who start using bioidentical hormones during the peri-menopausal period never lose the cardioprotective effect of estrogen as they continue to maintain adequate levels. It is the women who go through menopause and don't replace their hormones, who develop cardiovascular problems, such as heart attack and stroke. Replacing hormones in perimenopausal women isn't just about hot flashes and night sweats. It's about preventing heart attacks and strokes, maintaining youthful skin and hair, maintaining excellent energy levels, improving mood and outlook on life, improving libido and sexual function, preventing osteoporosis, and improving body composition and overall health. It's all about extending their health span for as long as possible. There is a difference in women who are in a comprehensive age-management program on hormone replacement therapy versus those who are not. It is obvious. You can see the difference the moment they come into a room.

Women in a comprehensive program with well-balanced hormones generally look younger and more vibrant, have better skin and hair, have a better outlook on life, and are more satisfied with their life. This is not surprising as they have better energy levels, feel better, and are able to maintain intimacy with their significant other. Many post-menopausal women I see, who are not on any type of program or hormone replacement therapy, simply look old. And the reality is they are. One of the things that keeps us young and healthy is our hormones. This is one of the theories as to the cause of aging. So, as our hormones decline more and more, we get older and feel older.

Women who go through menopause and do not maintain their hormones properly, in general, will not age well. Hormone replacement therapy in women if started early enough (within five years of menopause) will protect them from heart disease. As mentioned, and this is worth repeating, the most common cause of death in women after menopause is cardiovascular disease: heart attacks and strokes. It is not breast cancer. Hormone replacement therapy also alleviates the symptoms of menopause including hot flashes, night sweats, vaginal dryness, decreased libido, painful sexual intercourse, poor sleep, poor memory, and fuzzy thinking. It also helps maintain muscle mass and bone density.

Your hormones are extremely important in maintaining good health and in aging well, and hopefully you're a believer by now! Without them, we all would shrivel up, become frail and feeble, and eventually die.

So, it's not hard to see how some may call hormones "the fountain of youth." Hormones are not the fountain of youth, but they are very helpful in managing the aging process. The closest thing we have to the fountain of youth is how we live our lives—our lifestyle health habits. Clean, healthy eating with supplementation to fill in any holes in your diet, along with regular exercise with avoidance of alcohol and tobacco will expand your health span and your lifespan more than any one thing or pill. You are your own fountain of youth.

You can shorten or lengthen your life span and health span by how you lead your life. How does your future look to you?

CHAPTER 9

STRESS AND THE IMPACT ON YOUR BODY

How Well Do You Manage Stress?

Stress is ever-present in today's modern world. The pace of living has accelerated so much over the years that it's possible to never stop and smell the roses. The demands on our time have never been greater. With today's technology, people stay connected 24/7 and are bombarded with information overload. We are constantly being pulled in all directions. Many find it hard to get off the mouse wheel.

Stress is a significant factor to consider in an age-management program as it is one of the causes of accelerated aging. Many people don't even realize that they are under stress or are unaware of how that stress is impacting their body and their health. Chronic stress is associated with most chronic diseases, including diabetes and cardiovascular diseases, such as heart attack and stroke, as well as cancer.

I can usually tell if a patient is under stress by looking at their blood work and body composition scan. Unrecognized stress can be picked up in your blood work as an elevation of the stress hormone cortisol. When you are under stress, either acute or chronic, your body secretes cortisol. Chronically elevated cortisol can wreak havoc on your body. Often patients are surprised to see that their cortisol is elevated, not realizing that they have been under chronic stress. It is only after seeing their test results, in retrospect they realize that they have been feeling the effects of stress.

Chronic elevation of cortisol is deleterious to your body. It causes you to lose muscle mass and gain fat, the exact opposite of what we are trying to achieve in our age-management program. Rather than putting on muscle and losing fat, your muscles wither away, and you put on fat in all the wrong places, especially your belly. The loss of muscle mass can lead to sarcopenia which can lead to frailty and feebleness. The increase in belly fat increases chronic inflammation causing your body to deteriorate further. It's a downward spiral.

Chronically elevated cortisol increases your blood sugar, which can lead to insulin resistance and even diabetes. Diabetes is one of the best models we have of accelerated aging. Diabetics age faster than nondiabetics. Their health span is shorter, and they get more chronic diseases.

EXERCISE CAN REVERSE THE EFFECTS OF A STRESSFUL LIFE.

Chronic stress worsens chronic inflammation, which gradually eats away at your body. Elevated cortisol levels negatively impact your immune system making you more prone to colds, infections, and cancer. We all have heard stories of someone losing a spouse after many years of marriage; then six months later, the other spouse succumbs to cancer, heart attack, or pneumonia. This is a classic example of the immune system being suppressed by stress, allowing infection, inflammation, or cancer to overwhelm the body.

Stress can also impact cognitive function and is a risk factor for Alzheimer's and dementia.

A recent study from Wisconsin University School of Medicine revealed that stressful life experiences could age the brain by several years. Even one stressful event in life can influence later brain health. They showed that a larger number of life stress events was associated with poorer cognitive function later in life.

Eliminating and Managing Stress Is Key to Aging Well

The first step in reducing or eliminating stress is to recognize that it is there. You can't fix something until you know it is broken. Once you recognize the cause of your stress, you should do your best to eliminate it, or if it is impossible to eliminate, at least mitigate its effect on you. We have various tools available to us, including nutritional supplements to support the adrenal glands which produce cortisol, as well as meditation and biofeedback which have a calming effect. They stimulate the parasympathetic nervous system, which opposes the effects of the sympathetic nervous system. Stress causes an overstimulation of the sympathetic nervous system, which must be counterbalanced by the parasympathetic nervous system, thus bringing everything back in balance. Stress throws your body out of balance.

People who are under stress don't look healthy on the outside nor are they healthy on the inside. They may turn to addiction or alcohol and end up becoming even more unhealthy, compounding their problems. The way we live and age is all knitted together. I'm sure you've seen someone who can't seem to manage the stress in their lives properly and the way it has impacted them.

It's a commitment to pay attention to your emotional wellbeing to keep all parts of your life and body balanced and in working order. Stress management is a process of knowing yourself, your triggers, and your strengths and weaknesses.

Why Mindset Matters

Studies of centenarians show that one of their common traits is that they continue to socialize with others. Isolation is not a trait of centenarians. Isolation is not healthy. Humans were meant to be social as are parrots. Some studies conducted on African parrots have shown that parrots kept in isolation had shorter telomeres compared to parrots who had a companion. They aged faster in isolation. Telomeres are our cells' biologic timekeepers. Telomere length has been used as a marker of cellular aging. The longer your telomeres, the younger your cells are, and the younger you are.

Isolation can be toxic. Humans are social creatures. They need each other to thrive and survive. They derive energy, hope, comfort, ideas, and help from each other. Life is better and more satisfying if you can share it with other people. As humans, when we find ourselves in isolation, it can cause added stress and anxiety. When combined with poor lifestyle choices and poor diet, it will cause rapid aging.

Lifestyle changes can create stress if you're not prepared for them. When people get old, they often feel isolated as their friends die off or their kids go to college. It can be a small but significant process of stress that impacts their mindset. Knowing this, it may be important to take preventive measures in advance. How can you predict and alleviate the stress that comes with aging? As people age, they can feel helpless as their level of function declines, especially if mobility and ability are affected. That loss of independence can cause a massive decline in health as the body is overwhelmed by the physiologic effects of chronic stress. Proper planning can alleviate a lot of this stress.

Managing Stress

An excellent way to manage stress is to exercise. Not only does it help to burn fat and build muscle, but it releases endorphins, your feel-good hormones. Exercise has been shown in many studies to help with depression and anxiety and thus with stress. One of the best lifestyle choices you can make as you age is a commitment to increase your fitness goals daily so that you, too, can lose fat and build muscle. Don't listen to the stats about inevitably losing muscle every year.

It's possible to prevent age-related muscle loss and sarcopenia by doing resistance training regularly. It's never too late to reverse the trend. Most of the older people you see with sarcopenia from progressive muscle loss are that way because they did little to slow it down or reverse it by not doing weight training. The best way to keep your muscle mass and not lose it is to use it. The more you use it, the longer you will have it, and the bigger it will be.

As humans age, often appetite declines and protein consumption decreases. Proteins contain amino acids, the building blocks of muscle. Without protein, you will not be able to build muscle. If your diet is poor and instead of protein you eat the wrong things such as processed carbs, you will accumulate belly fat instead of building muscle. A buildup of abdominal fat will lead to chronic inflammation and excess estrogen; add to that the decline in testosterone that occurs with aging, and you will find yourself battling sarcopenia, too. That's why you see some people with low daily caloric intake still have large bellies and skinny arms and legs. They are eating the wrong foods and not exerting adequately. With blood sugar spikes, lack of exercise, lack of protein, lack of nutrition, and lack of hormones, you will get muscle loss and a distended abdomen. If you see this in yourself already, it's time to improve your nutrition and get to work building muscle! You can work on strengthening your core and muscles daily by increasing your protein and supplement intake and committing to a regular exercise routine to build muscle and shrink your belly. The best option, of course, is a formal age-management program to target your specific goals, strengths, and weaknesses and optimize your hormones so that you can function at your best.

When you don't do anything to take care of your health, you significantly decrease your life expectancy. If you can reduce the stress on your mind and your body, you will age well. Stress, like diabetes, can cause accelerated aging. It all comes down to diet and lifestyle. Reduce stress, improve your diet and nutrition, adopt healthy lifestyle choices, and make a commitment to decelerate the aging process!

CHAPTER 10

DIAGNOSIS, PLANNING, AND EXECUTION

In medicine, you must have the right diagnosis, or the plan you create and execute will fail. Think of the importance of a proper diagnosis as the foundation for getting healthy and strong. To get the right diagnosis, a doctor has to spend a lot of time with the patient. It can't be a drive-by experience. As a physician, I learn so much by observing, listening, and spending time with my patients and asking the right questions. You really have to listen.

My first step in determining a diagnosis is interviewing my patients. I go way back in time through their entire history. When did they first notice the problem or symptom? Often, they don't realize that their current complaints are related to something that happened a long time ago. If you take a careful look at their history, you may find that an injury that happened fifteen years ago is having an impact on their current complaints. You really must interview the patient in depth, find out when the problem may have been in its infancy, and then, by asking the right questions, you can determine how it progressed.

Some patients are good historians while others are not. It is the poor historians that make my job more difficult as I may not have all the relevant information that I need to come up with the correct diagnosis. The more information that you have, the better and more accurate a diagnosis you can make. Sometimes what may seem like a sudden event in their lives was caused by something that occurred many years in the past but was left untreated, such as a physical or sports injury or a minor car accident. What seemed trivial at the time may have had some real consequences for the future.

The next thing that I look at is demeanor. A great doctor observes all things, not just what the patient is saying. Are they anxious, are they upset, are they nervous, or are they an introvert? Body language can tell you so much about what a patient is going through. If they are chronically anxious and stressed, they are going to have huge spikes in their cortisol levels and even adrenaline and norepinephrine (stress hormones), and that can create a whole host of health problems.

The third thing I look at is their skin, hair, and eyes and how healthy they appear. Someone healthy will have bright eyes, glowing skin, great hair, and lots of energy. Someone who is having medical issues will not look good and often much older. Their color will be poor. Their skin is thin, dry, sagging, and pale. Their hair is thinning and dull. They may have dark circles under their eyes. They will look tired and worn out, drained of energy.

Prior to my seeing them, I have my patients fill out a thirty-four-page detailed questionnaire about their health and all aspects of their life including health, habits, family, lifestyle, diet, exercise, work, stressors, challenges, accomplishments, and so forth. You name it, we cover it.

An extensive blood work analysis is performed before their first visit to look at their various biomarkers of health, including fifteen different hormones as well as markers of inflammation. After reviewing the lab work, we can tell just how much inflammation is happening in their bodies and how well their body is handling sugars, carbs, and fats. We look at their metabolism, kidney, liver, blood cells, and blood chemistry as well as some vitamin levels.

We look at the health of their blood vessels. Is the lining of their arteries inflamed and thickened? Do they have cholesterol plaque accumulating in their arteries? Are they closing off slowly? If so, they may be at risk for stroke or heart attack. We also look at how well their brain is working. Are there any cognitive or memory issues? Is their brain working more slowly than normal? Is their processing speed and reaction time off? Is their attention and mental focus off? All this can be tested and may detect a problem before it is clinically apparent. Think of it as an early warning system for dementia and Alzheimer's disease.

One of my favorite tests is the Lunar iDXA scan. With this sophisticated machine, which scans your entire body while you lay on the scan table, we can measure exactly how much fat, lean muscle, and bone you have to the gram. Not only does it show you these values for your body as a whole, but it also shows you these parameters for different body regions, such as your stomach, hips, trunk, arms, and legs. Looking at the left and right sides as well as combined. We can tell how your fat and muscle are distributed and how much of each you have. We can calculate the percent of body fat not only for your body as a whole but for each body region. By performing these scans on a regular basis throughout the year, we can see if you are making progress and getting the changes in your body composition that you are looking for. We can even tell if your bones are soft and whether you have osteopenia or osteoporosis.

Good health doesn't happen by accident. You have to pay attention and be proactive. You have to participate. This is not a spectator program. You have to avoid poor lifestyle habits and institute a healthy lifestyle plan and keep at it. If you don't pay attention, you may go in the wrong direction.

Poor health doesn't happen overnight. It develops slowly over the years with the slow and gradual decay of our bodies as a consequence of the many poor choices we made in what we put into our bodies and how well we exercised our bodies and our minds. Eventually this catches up to us and we have to assess the damage.

It takes time to create an accurate picture of a patient and to derive at a correct diagnosis. This is hard to do if not impossible in a fifteen-minute office visit.

For good outcomes, it is all about making the correct diagnosis. This is true for age management as well as neurosurgery. In my neurosurgical practice, I often see patients with spine-related problems. They may report complaints of arm or leg numbness and weakness with difficulty walking. Some may have pain, others not. Some are even in wheelchairs. Complaints of this sort can be caused by problems anywhere in the nervous system, including the brain, spine, or spinal cord. Even a peripheral nerve problem can be at fault. The way to figure out what is going on is to do a thorough history, perform a good neurological exam, obtain appropriate diagnostic testing including scans, and then review the scans and all available information. It is only then that you can formulate a rational treatment plan.

THE ORGANS OF YOUR BODY THAT HAVE THE MOST CONCENTRATION OF TESTOSTERONE RECEPTORS ARE YOUR HEART AND YOUR BRAIN. THERE MUST BE A GOOD REASON FOR THAT; GOD DOESN'T MAKE MISTAKES.

Some problems can be corrected with surgery, others not. If a surgical treatment plan is decided, it is important to review the preoperative scans carefully before surgery to see where the potential trouble spots might be in order avoid complications and optimize outcomes. Where is the pathology? What is it harming? How do I get it out without damaging the brain, spinal cord, or nerves? Where are problems likely to be encountered? How do I stay out of trouble? What is the safest, most effective, least invasive surgery that I can do?

I follow a similar approach in my age-management practice. After a careful review of the history, physical exam, diagnostics, and testing, I determine what the strengths and weaknesses of my patient are and then formulate a treatment plan. The execution of that plan, in this case, rests with the patient. It is up to them to follow the treatment plan. I can coach them and advise them along the way, but it is up to them to incorporate the plan into their everyday life if they want to get the results they desire.

Ultimately, your health is your responsibility. You can change your life and slow down or even reverse the aging process with careful planning and execution. Sometimes it takes the intervention of someone like me to be your health coach and advisor in much the same way an elite athlete needs a coach! The best of the best always have coaches to keep them at their optimum.

I'm in the business of helping people correct poor lifestyle habits. We can measure their progress with regular blood tests and body composition scans. I can usually tell well ahead of time before even seeing the patient in follow-up, if they have been sticking to the plan simply by reviewing their lab and scan results. We usually do this quarterly to pick up problems early in their infancy before they become clinical problems.

Are You Aging Well?

We want you to age as slowly as possible. We want you to be optimal and not just average. Have you ever read the "average recommended daily allowances" description on a vitamin box? What if you have a deficiency and you need more than the average amount? Everybody is different. I doubt you're average.

Hormones are important for good health. When we deliver the right mix of hormones, we can literally change someone's physical and emotional wellbeing. You have to follow the program carefully, making each step a priority. If you do, then you will see huge strides in your health, and the positive changes in your body will happen. But there are also individuals who will never see changes because they unknowingly sabotage their progress with poor eating habits. You simply cannot out-exercise a bad diet. If you don't eat cleanly, you will never get optimal results.

Something that I have noticed over the years is that there are people who don't want to follow all of our advice. There are people who participate in the program and don't want to exercise. Others don't want to change their diet. Despite having some patients who don't use the program to its fullest potential, I have never seen anyone *not* get better and improve their lives at least to some degree. Some positive change is better than no change at all.

If you are blaming time as the reason as to why you can't be healthier, then you are using the wrong reason. If you want to live longer and time is the reason why you say you can't work out, then you should work out even more. Because that is what will prolong your life. I'm a busy neurosurgeon, and I don't have much free time, but I always make exercise a priority. I exercise six times a week even if I am exhausted after a long surgical day. What you make a priority, you will do.

If you want dramatic results, you have to put in the effort. You have to do everything in the plan. Success isn't driven by how you feel. Success is driven by what you do. Good outcomes are a result of the correct diagnosis, careful planning, and diligent execution.

CHAPTER 11

NUTRITION AND SUPPLEMENTS

Nutrition Is Everything.

Your body thrives on healthy foods and requires certain nutrients to function properly. To reach peak performance, eat as clean and as simple as possible. Eat whole, real, natural, and preferably organic food. The closer it is to the way it came out of the ground, tree, or bush the better. The less processed, the better. The more a food is changed from its natural form, the less nutritious it is.

Eat Clean

Eating the wrong things can make you old fast. There are certain foods, like sugar and processed carbohydrates, that can accelerate aging and therefore should be avoided at all costs. While we all love sugar because of its sweet taste, sugar is your enemy. It makes you old. It's almost like the Trojan horse. You put it into your body, and it tastes good and makes you feel good. In fact, it tastes so good that you want more, but in excess, it begins to degrade your body. Preparing your own meals is best as you know exactly what you are getting. When you don't prepare your own food, you have no idea how much sugar, fat, and salt is being added, and what you don't know can ultimately hurt you and, in some cases, kill you. People are eating out more and more out of convenience, but there are hidden sugars and preservatives in processed and prepared foods that you would not consume if you prepared a clean meal yourself at home. For optimal health and to function at your highest level, prepare the majority of your meals at home. Your mind and body will love you for it.

The Simpler the Food the Better

When you're dining out, you may think you know what's on the menu, but you don't really know what additives they are putting in your food. Studies have compared similar meals made at home versus eaten at a restaurant. The meals made at home were in general far healthier than their counterparts in a restaurant because restaurants tend to use a lot more added sugar, salt, and fat than you would at home.

Unless you prepare your meal yourself, it's hard to control what goes into it. The food may have lots of hidden sugar in the form of high glycemic carbohydrates, which get broken down into sugar. Anything that gets broken down into sugar results in a blood sugar spike, which triggers the release of insulin. In the presence of insulin, any sugar (glucose) that is not metabolized for energy is converted to triglycerides and stored as fat. In the presence of insulin, it is impossible to mobilize fat stores and use fat for fuel.

You can only store fat. In the presence of insulin, as your blood sugar drops, you become hungry again in an attempt to raise your blood sugar, so you eat again. If what you eat again is another high glycemic carbohydrate, such as bread, white rice, or a potato, you spike your blood sugar once again, which spikes your insulin, which converts more sugar to fat, which makes your belly even larger. By eating high glycemic carbohydrates, you are essentially directly feeding your fat stores, and until you stop, you will get bigger and bigger. No amount of exercise will undo this damage. Only a lifestyle change to a high-protein, low-saturated-fat, low-glycemic diet will make a difference. Only then will exercise have an impact. Fat doesn't make you fat; sugar makes you fat, and it does this by way of insulin.

Let us also not forget advanced glycation end products (AGE). Glycation is when the sugar in your bloodstream attaches to proteins to form a molecule known as advanced glycation end products. These products have been associated with aging and the development of chronic diseases such as diabetes, Alzheimer's disease, and atherosclerosis.

Take action to control the variables that you are able to systemize and control easily. Two of the most important things that you control in life are exercise and diet. We control when and how much we move, and we control what goes into our mouths. When it comes to your health, there are things that you can do to optimize it, and some things that you have no control over. Concentrate on the things you can change. One of those variables is nutritional supplementation.

Why Do We Need Supplements?

In a perfect world, we would not need supplements. But as I said before, we don't live in a perfect world. Our bodies are constantly being stressed. We are exposed to free radicals, oxidation, inflammation, advanced glycation end products, radiation, and toxins. Our DNA, cell membranes, and cell organelles are constantly at risk of being damaged. We need nutritional supplementation to prevent this damage, especially to our DNA and telomeres.

Nutritional supplementation can help with every aspect of aging from the physical to mental decline. Nutritional supplementation works from the inside out and can help to fill holes and deficiencies left by our imperfect diets. None of us eat perfectly. It is virtually impossible for all of us to get all of the daily vitamins, minerals, and trace elements that we need in today's modern world, where our soils have become nutritionally depleted over the decades. In fact only about 10 percent of adults meet the federal recommendations for daily intake of fruit and vegetables. A CDC Morbidity and Mortality Weekly Report published November 2017 reported that in 2015 only 9 percent of adults met the recommended guidelines for vegetable intake and only 12 percent met the intake guidelines for fruit. Thus 90 percent of the population is likely nutritionally deficient and should be on at least a broad spectrum multivitamin such as *Vitamere Anti Aging* or *Vitamere-Ultra Anti Aging* (patents pending). These provide not only the usual vitamins, minerals and trace elements of a multipurpose, broad spectrum multivitamin, but they also have added ingredients that have been shown in the scientific literature to promote cellular and DNA health as well as promote and in many cases increase the size of your telomeres thus reversing cellular aging. You can think of this as a form of cellular rejuvenation or cellular defense. Protect your cells and your DNA and they will live longer and as a result you will live longer and healthier.

Supplementation Impacts Telomeres

Telomeres are the cellular time keepers that determine the rate at which you age. The longer your telomeres, the "younger" your cells and the healthier you are. The human body has a protective enzyme known as telomerase that helps to rebuild, protect, repair, and lengthen your telomeres. Recent research shows that there are specific nutrients that stimulate your body to produce the enzyme telomerase.

We now have a scientifically validated way to support telomeres and have them remain more youthful for a longer period of time. One way is via supplementation. I take a nutraceutical product called *Vitamere Ultra Anti Aging* that I developed and began taking in 2012. Prior to that, between 2008 and 2012, I was taking a regular multivitamin without the special ingredients that I incorporated in *Vitamere Ultra*. This had a profound effect in reversing cellular aging in my body, as measured by mean telomere length. My mean telomere length (MTL) went from that of a thirty-nine year old in 2012 to that of a twenty year old in 2017. I was literally able to reverse cellular aging in my body as measured by MTL.

Nothing else had changed in my age-management program between the two time periods—2008–2012 and 2012–2017—other than my substituting *Vitamere Ultra Anti Aging* for the old multivitamin that I was taking. My diet, exercise, and lifestyle were otherwise identical both before and after *Vitamere Ultra Anti Aging*. The only variable was *Vitamere Ultra Anti Aging*.

A combined 402 peer-reviewed scientific studies support the ingredients in *Vitamere Anti Aging* and *Vitamere Ultra Anti Aging*. These ingredients help to support and maintain telomeres, our cellular time keepers. Telomeres have been recognized as excellent biomarkers of how well we are aging. They are a proxy for cellular aging. You are only as old as your telomeres. Keep them young. How long would you like *your* telomeres to be?

THE BRAIN AND HEART ARE ORGANS THAT NEED TESTOSTERONE TO FUNCTION PROPERLY. THEY ALSO NEED NUTRIENTS FROM FOOD AND BLOOD CIRCULATION FROM EXERCISE.

What Is a Nutraceutical?

The term *nutraceutical* was coined in the 1990s by Dr. Stephen DeFelice, who defined it as "any substance that is a food or a part of a food that provides medical or health benefits, including the prevention and treatment of disease." Health Canada defines nutraceutical as "a product isolated or purified from foods, and generally sold in medicinal forms not usually associated with food and demonstrated to have a physiological benefit or provide protection against chronic disease." Based upon these definitions, a nutraceutical could include vitamins, minerals, herbs, and other natural substances.

If you've ever worked out in a gym or grown up around fitness buffs, you've noticed that they have one thing in common besides lifting weights, and that's supplementation. It's not uncommon to see bodybuilders or fit and healthy people consistently performing their routine in the gym every day with a shaker of what looks like a milky-colored, cloudy water, filled with amino acids or protein powder. It's a form of supplementation that helps them repair and build their muscles.

DIETARY SUPPLEMENTATION IS CRITICAL TO MAINTAINING HEALTHY LEVELS.

Our bodies need the proper fuel to perform at peak function and often after testing blood; we discover that these nutrients and hormones are depleted. It's not uncommon to discover a vitamin or hormonal deficiency such as low levels of thyroid, testosterone, and vitamin D. Even vitamin B12 can be low.

According to the Council for Responsible Nutrition's (CRN):

The Dietary Supplement Health and Education Act of 1994 (DSHEA) defines dietary supplements as products intended to supplement the diet. According to DSHEA, dietary supplements may contain vitamins, minerals, herbs or other botanicals, amino acids, other dietary substances, or combinations or extracts of any of these "dietary ingredients."

Supplementation is different for everyone but may involve individual or combination vitamin and mineral supplements, herbal supplements, certain limited types of hormones (e.g., melatonin, DHEA), biological substances (e.g., glucosamine sulfate, chondroitin sulfate), and specialty products. By focusing on the right mix of individualized supplementation, we can promote energy metabolism, reduce the effects of stress, and increase weight loss.

Sports performance is enhanced with legal supplementation, which is why you see athletes supplementing their diets with protein powders, vitamins, shakes, and several other carefully fine-tuned combinations. When they work with their coaches and medical team to tweak their specific formula, they've tested and retested their blood to determine what specific nutrients they're lacking and how to provide it best. Athletes, especially, are prone to depletion of certain vitamins and minerals through training and therefore must be conscious of exactly how their bodies are processing food and liquids and where they specifically need supplementation. But this is true for everyone—the athlete and the average individual as well!

The Nutrient Content of Our Food

An examination of our food supply over a ninety-year period does not show a substantial improvement in the nutrient level of foods in general; in fact, the data suggests the opposite. This is evident in the blood tests we see weekly in our office with patients often depleted in key vitamins such as B and D.

Despite improvements in agricultural techniques, which have improved crop yield, from 1909 to 1994 a decrease in the levels of vital nutrients has occurred. The vitamin B12 levels in foods decreased about 5 percent, magnesium decreased about 3 percent, zinc decreased about 3 percent, and potassium decreased about 7 percent. Of course, on the face of it, a 3–7 percent decrease of vital nutrients doesn't sound too bad. On the other hand, this is a decrease of nutrients across our food supply.

An examination of individual crops can reveal a more severe decrease. As a matter of fact, a review of some research about growing conditions, agricultural technologies, and nutrient content of the soil can reveal just how significantly these issues can affect the nutrient levels in some crops. Since everything we eat impacts our aging, it's worthwhile to understand how our nation's food supply and production can affect our individual lives.

Instead of debating organic versus nonorganic foods, it's best to truly understand where food comes from, how it's produced, and how what you're eating is impacting your body, blood, aging, and telomeres. With regular blood glucose testing, you can determine what impact your diet is having on your body. With the knowledge we gain from your blood tests, we can design a specific program that's tailored just for you to slow down or even reverse aging. This is what we do in my office in our age-management program.

Understanding Growing Conditions and Crop Nutrient Levels

In one study, the properties of some extensively cultivated sunflower seed varieties and their oils were investigated between two years of crops in Turkey (sunflower seeds are one of the goods that Turkey exports to the USA). Analysis revealed that the growing conditions significantly affected the fatty acid composition of sunflower varieties studied. For example, the essential unsaturated fatty acid linoleic acid levels decreased across the board approximately 20 percent. Also, vitamin E levels (alpha-tocopherol) remained constant in some instances; in other cases, vitamin E levels decreased by nearly 20 percent. When you consider that the USDA rates sunflower seeds as the number one non-enriched food source of vitamin E and rates them as the number two non-enriched food source of polyunsaturated fatty acids, such a discrepancy is problematic. What if an individual had integrated sunflower seeds into his or her diet in an attempt to help fulfill the requirements of these nutrients, but the actual levels were 20 percent less?

In another study, the growing conditions of lettuce affected calcium content of the lettuce leaves. Developing lettuce leaves that could freely open out from the head were compared to lettuce leaves that were enclosed within a developing head. The use of lettuce enclosures is not unusual in agriculture. In any case, the lettuce that could freely open without enclosure developed normally, whereas lettuce developing with enclosure had a calcium deficiency.

As a matter of fact, the lettuce *without* enclosures provided 300 percent more calcium than the enclosed lettuce. How food is produced impacts the nutrients the food provides. We can shortcut success by being educated about our food. Why wouldn't we want to know more about the greatest gift we've been given—our health? When patients are educated, they have the power to create massive change through the right choices. I've seen patients make a complete turnaround in their health simply by becoming educated about food, nutrients, and sugar. Some even grow their own food!

Agricultural Technologies and Crop Nutrient Levels

In addition to growing conditions, agricultural technologies can also affect crop nutrient levels. Analysis of tomato nutrition has demonstrated that certain agriculture technologies can increase the content of vitamin A and niacin. This result sounds positive, yet at the same time, vitamin C and E contents decreased by 2 percent and 13 percent, respectively. Likewise, among the minerals that were analyzed in tomatoes, many increased in content, but seven decreased. Hopefully not too many people were eating these tomatoes together with Turkish sunflower seeds to boost their vitamin E levels.

Carbon dioxide (CO_2) enrichment is a method used to affect the yield of lettuce and radishes grown in controlled environments. In one study, these crops were grown both in the field and in a controlled chamber environment where CO_2 enrichment was used. The levels of certain minerals differed between field- and chamber-grown crops, including changes in the calcium and phosphorus (P) contents of radish and lettuce leaves, resulting in reduced calcium-phosphorus ratio for chamber-grown materials. Furthermore, total dietary fiber content was much higher in the field-grown plant material. Consequently, even though CO_2 enrichment can improve crop yield, it is not necessarily advantageous with regard to crop nutrition.

Nutrient Content of the Soil and Crop Nutrient Levels

Aside from growing conditions and agricultural technologies, there is the simple fact that the nutrient content of foods can be directly related to the nutrient content of the soil in which they were grown. For example, the selenium content of plants, in particular cereal grains, is strongly influenced by the quantity of biologically available selenium in the soil in which they grow, that is, by their geographical origin. As a result, it should not be too much of a surprise that, according to the USDA, the selenium content of fruits and vegetables is normally very low.

Healthy Choices

Another issue is that the actual diet we choose to eat may not be very good. It might, in fact, be harmful. There's so much available to each one of us on a daily basis from donut drive-through to Asian food to all sorts of fast-food restaurants, to pizza, and to food brought into the office. Some people make the mistake of believing that the healthy fast-food chains are healthy, or that the salads in restaurants are packed with healthy ingredients. Some of the salads in restaurants top 1,000 calories each and are actually packed with extra cheese, fats, dressing, and sugars! Be careful what you put in your mouth.

What constitutes a good diet? According to the USDA, it's MyPlate. In June 2011, MyPlate replaced the previous dietary guidelines known as MyPyramid. According to the USDA, "MyPlate is part of a larger communications initiative based on *2010 Dietary Guidelines for Americans* to help consumers make better food choices. MyPlate is designed to *remind* Americans to eat healthfully; it is not intended to change consumer behavior alone."

The MyPlate icon depicts five food groups using a mealtime place setting of a plate and a glass. It is divided into sections of approximately 30 percent grains, 30 percent vegetables, 20 percent fruits, and 20 percent protein, accompanied by a smaller

circle representing dairy, such as a glass of low-fat/nonfat milk
or a yogurt cup.

Former First Lady Michelle Obama explained the basic ratio-
nale for the switch from MyPyramid to MyPlate when MyPlate
was unveiled:

> Parents don't have the time to measure exactly three ounces
> of chicken or to look up how much rice or broccoli is in a
> serving. But we do have time to look at our kids' plates. And
> if they're eating proper portions, as long as half of their meal
> is fruits and vegetables alongside their lean proteins, whole
> grains, and low-fat dairy, then we're good. It's as simple as
> that.

MyPlate also recommends:

- Make half your plate fruits and vegetables;
- Switch to 1 percent or skim milk;
- Make at least half your grains whole;
- Vary your protein food choices;
- Control your portions while still enjoying food; and
- Reduce sodium and sugar intakes.

Nevertheless, MyPlate is not without its critics. Walter Willett,
PhD, Chair of the Department of Nutrition for Harvard School
of Public Health (HSPH), criticized MyPlate, saying, "Unfortunately, like the earlier US Department of Agriculture Pyramids,
MyPlate mixes science with the influence of powerful agricultural
interests, which is not the recipe for healthy eating."

Consequently, HSPH released their own adjusted and more
detailed version of MyPlate, called the Harvard Healthy Eating Plate. Harvard's plate features a higher ratio of vegetables
to fruit, adds healthy oils to the recommendation, and balances

healthy protein and whole grains as equal quarters of the plate, along with recommending water and suggesting sparing dairy consumption.

Whether following MyPlate or the Harvard Healthy Eating Plate, these dietary guidelines don't translate into actual benefits if individuals don't follow the recommendations. So, let's examine how many actually adhere to dietary recommendations. Eating habits vary from country to country, but in America, here are the facts:

Report Card on American Diets

The diets of most Americans need to improve, according to the USDA, indicated by the Healthy Eating Index (HEI). During 1999–2000, the diets of most people (74 percent) needed improvement. Only 10 percent of the population had a good diet; 16 percent had a poor diet. Unfortunately, the diet quality of Americans, as assessed by the most recent HEI in 2010 (which assessed 2007–2008 diets), did not change, with three exceptions. Scores declined for sodium and increased for whole fruit and empty calories. In both 2001–2002 and 2007–2008, HEI-2010 scores were below the maximum possible score for all components, except for total protein foods. In 2007–2008, scores for greens and beans, whole grains, fatty acids, sodium, and empty calories were below 50 percent of their maximums. Scores for the remaining components were also substantially below their maximums (57 percent to 72 percent) in most cases. HEI-2010 researchers concluded, "The diet quality of Americans is far from optimal and, according to the HEI-2010 total score, did not improve overall between 2001–02 and 2007–08."

Nutrient Intake of Americans

So, for the 10 percent of Americans who are following dietary guidelines, will they receive 100 percent of the recommended daily intake (RDI) for micronutrients (vitamins and minerals)?

According to the goals of nutrient intake established by the USDA, comparing the nutritional goals for Americans to the nutrient content of foods consumed in a 2,000-calorie-per-day diet, there will be insufficient amounts of vitamin D, vitamin E, choline, magnesium (for men only), and potassium. Imagine that— *even if you follow dietary guidelines, you won't be reaching 100 percent of your nutrient intake goals.* That's because of the nutrient content of our foods. Data from the USDA shows that the vitamin content of foods has indeed changed—and not for the better.

This decline is made even worse when you consider that this includes foods that are already enriched with vitamins. Furthermore, the most recent National Health and Nutrition Examination Survey (NHANES) indicates that:

- Vitamin B6, iron and vitamin D are the three nutrients with the highest prevalence of deficiency.

- Vitamin C and vitamin B12 are nutrients with intermediate prevalence of deficiency.

- Older adults were more likely to be vitamin B12 deficient.

- Men were more likely to be vitamin C deficient compared to women.

- Non-Hispanic black and Mexican-American (12 percent) people were more likely to be vitamin D deficient compared to non-Hispanic white people.

This is becoming increasingly common knowledge for those educated in age management. Vitamin deficiency is something many adults are aware of if they've taken care of their bodies and gotten their blood tested. The conclusion is that supplementation is absolutely necessary to a vital life. You can live without it—but not at your best.

One study addressed this issue of nutrition by examining the nutrient content of four popular diet plans: two different versions of the *Atkins* diet, *The South Beach Diet*, and *the DASH diet*.

The analysis determined that each of the four popular diet plans failed to provide minimum recommended daily intake (RDI) sufficiency for twenty-seven of the micronutrients (vitamins and minerals) analyzed.

Further analysis of the 4 diets found that an average intake of 27,575 calories would be required to achieve sufficiency in all 27 micronutrients! Six micronutrients (biotin, vitamin D, vitamin E, chromium, iodine, and molybdenum) were identified as consistently low or nonexistent in all 4 diet plans. Clearly, eating a different diet plan isn't likely to improve your dietary report card where nutrients are concerned.

Dietary Supplements: A Nutrition Insurance Policy

Since people are clearly not getting an adequate amount of nutrients from their diet, this would seem to make a strong case for using dietary supplements as a "nutrition insurance policy." In fact, the American Medical Association Journal (*JAMA*), stated:

> Most people do not consume an optimal amount of all vitamins by diet alone. Pending strong evidence of effectiveness from randomized trials, it appears prudent for all adults to take vitamin supplements.

Considering that the AMA has not traditionally been in favor of the routine use of dietary supplements, this is truly a landmark recommendation on their part. Another statement made in the same *JAMA* study helps to shed some light on why the change of position:

> Vitamin deficiency syndromes such as scurvy and beriberi are uncommon in Western societies. However, suboptimal intake of some vitamins, above levels, causing classic vitamin deficiency, is a risk factor for chronic diseases and common in the general population, especially the elderly.

Apparently, the suboptimal intake of nutrients was significant enough to lead the AMA to the conclusion that supplementation is recommended for the general population. Marginal deficiencies appear to be far more widespread and can cause a variety of nonspecific symptoms while they weaken the body's defenses against serious illnesses.

So now that we've established the need for dietary supplements, the next question is how much of the essential vitamins and minerals, like folate, vitamin A, or calcium, are really needed every day to be healthy? Some would say that the RDAs for vitamins and minerals are appropriate. Yet other nutrition experts consider the RDA to be inadequate. To assess this divergence in opinion, let's examine governmental dietary allowances and standards in America alone, starting with the history of the RDAs.

Recommended Daily Allowances

For more than fifty years, the Food and Nutrition Board of the National Academy of Sciences (FNB) has been reviewing nutrition research and defining nutrient requirements for healthy people, referred to as the Recommended Dietary Allowances or RDA. When the RDAs were created in 1941, their primary goal was to prevent diseases caused by nutrient deficiencies. They were originally intended to evaluate and plan for the nutritional adequacy of groups, for example, the armed forces and children in school lunch programs, rather than to determine individuals' nutrient needs.

But, because the RDAs were essentially the only nutrient values available, they began to be used in ways other than the intended use. Health professionals often used RDAs to size-up the diets of their individual patients or clients. Statistically speaking, RDAs would prevent deficiency diseases in 97 percent of a population, but there was no scientific basis that RDAs would meet the needs of a single person. This was true even though there were 18 versions of the RDA, each for various age groups for infants, children, males, and females (including separate RDAs for during

THE DIETS OF MOST AMERICANS NEED TO IMPROVE. THIS IS TRUE IN MOST PARTS OF THE WORLD AS WELL, AS WE GROW AND DEVELOP AND BECOME A GLOBAL SOCIETY THAT HAS ACCESS TO EVERYTHING WE WANT—INCLUDING A LOT OF FAST FOODS.

pregnancy and lactation), and despite the fact that all of these versions were revised several times.

It was evident that the RDAs were not addressing individual needs, and new science needed to be included. Therefore, the Food and Nutrition Board sought to re-define nutrient requirements and develop specific nutrient recommendations for indi-viduals, as well as for groups. Along with these changes, concepts such as tolerable upper intakes and adequate intakes emerged to meet individual needs better.

How RDAs Became DRIs

In 1993, the Food and Nutrition Board put the RDA revision process into motion. Not only did the definition of RDAs change, but three new values were also created: The Estimated Average Requirement (EAR), the Adequate Intake (AI), and the Tolerable Upper Intake Level (UL). All four values are collectively known as Dietary Reference Intakes or DRIs. The first report of the DRI Committee was released in 1997 and focused on calcium, vitamin D, phosphorus, magnesium, and fluoride. The second report on thiamin, riboflavin, niacin, vitamin B6, folate, vitamin B12, pan-tothenic acid, biotin, and choline was released in spring 1998. Future reports will be published in the next few years.

The US RDA and Daily Values

Prior to the development of the DRIs, in 1973, the Food and Drug Administration established a new standard called the

United States Recommended Daily Allowances (US RDA) for use in nutrition labeling. The US RDA replaced the Minimum Daily Requirements (MDR), which had been used since 1941 in the labeling of food and dietary supplements. The US RDA was deemed to be the amount of various nutrients needed by healthy people plus an additional 30 to 50 percent to allow for individual variations. For example, if the 1 milligram of vitamin B1 was deemed to be adequate, then increasing it by 50 percent to 1.5 mg was considered to allow for individual variations.

Although a "one size fits all" nutrient standard does not really seem to be the best way to establish the nutrient needs for a diverse population, the existence of a standard was necessary for labeling. It would not be practical to include all eighteen versions of the RDA on the label of a prepared food or dietary supplement.

Then, because of the Nutritional Labeling and Education Act (NLEA), a new standard, called the "Daily Value," was created. At the risk of confusing everyone, the Daily Value was based on another new standard, called the Reference Daily Intakes (RDI). Actually, the RDI wasn't really new; it was basically the same as the US RDA, just with a few more nutrients included.

Disagreement by Other Nutrition Experts

As stated earlier, other nutrition experts disagree that the RDA/RDIs are an appropriate guideline for vitamin and mineral supplementation. The basic argument is that the RDA/RDIs do not really reflect the amount of a nutrient necessary to promote good health and stave off common diseases (e.g., coronary heart disease, cancer, etc.), but rather are the amount of a vitamin or mineral necessary to prevent classic nutrient deficiency disease states such as scurvy (vitamin C deficiency) or beriberi (vitamin B1 deficiency).

What's all this mean for you and your family?

Although intended to prevent nutritional deficiency diseases, the RDA is often used, incorrectly, as the optimum nutrient recommendation for a particular individual. RDAs do not take into account the effects of lifestyle (stress, smoking, etc.), nor do they consider nutritional needs associated with other disease processes (AIDS, cancer, etc.). The question of what the optimal dosages are for various vitamins and minerals boils down to the individual. Many nutrition studies research the specific effects of individual nutrients. However, nutrition study results often do not look at long-term effects or at effects on other nutrients or other systems in the body. (Dr. T. M. Culp)

These sentiments are echoed by renowned naturopathic physician Dr. Michael Murray:

A tremendous amount of scientific research indicates that the "optimal" level for many nutrients, especially the so-called antioxidant nutrients like vitamins C and E, beta-carotene and selenium may be much higher than their current RDAs. The RDAs focus on the prevention of nutritional deficiencies in population groups only; they do not define "optimal" intake for an individual. Other factors the RDAs do not adequately consider are environmental and lifestyle factors that can destroy vitamins and bind minerals. For example, even the Food and Nutrition Board acknowledges that smokers require at least twice as much vitamin C as non-smokers, but what about other nutrients and smoking? And what about the effects of alcohol consumption, food additives, heavy metals (lead, mercury, etc.), carbon monoxide, and other chemicals associated with our modern society that are known to interfere with nutrient function? Dealing with hazards of modern living may be another reason why many people take supplements.

The late nutritionist Shari Lieberman, PhD, author of *The Real Vitamin & Mineral Book,* had this to say about the RDI:

As it currently stands, the RDA is a limited concept, the meaning and usefulness of which are being questioned even by the experts who are responsible for establishing and maintaining it. In today's world, the RDIs are, with a few exceptions, the nutritional equivalent of the minimum wage. They are probably high enough to keep you alive—although even this is open to question. But they do not appear high enough to allow you to enjoy the best quality of life. And why should you not strive for the best?

Optimal Daily Intake

Perhaps the most significant commentaries disagreeing with the RDA/RDIs as a standard for dietary supplementation are the results of published research which demonstrates a clear benefit when consuming higher levels of vitamins and minerals. For the purposes of this discussion and also because it is a more accurate description, let's refer to these higher levels as the optimal daily intake (ODITI), a term coined by Dr. Lieberman.

Ultimately, I believe that each individual patient who walks into my office should be tested to understand their baseline for where they are nutritionally and where they need to be. You've only got one body—let's do this right! If you can't afford to get your blood tested regularly, at the very least you should be taking supplements.

The Three Supplements Everyone Should Take

Research has clearly shown that nutrition plays a significant role in determining our state of health and our susceptibility to many diseases. It has been estimated that *every year* there are:

- 14 million cases of preventable heart disease;
- 1.2 million preventable cases of cancer;

- More than half a million preventable strokes; and

- 2,500 babies born with neural tube defects that could have been prevented by a simple vitamin.

Disease prevention can reduce health care costs as well as lessen the personal burden of disease. For example, improving nutritional practices could potentially delay the onset of cardiovascular disease, stroke, and osteoporosis by 5 years, thus saving $89 billion in health care costs *annually*. While the overall improvement of dietary habits is the focus of much research on promoting health and preventing disease, we have seen from the previous discussion that Americans as a whole continue to employ poor dietary practices and have an inadequate intake of nutrients. This has led many scientists and healthcare professionals to recognize that dietary supplements may play an increasingly important role.

This leads to the question, which supplements should people take to help promote good health and at what doses? Vitamins? Minerals? Herbs? Nutraceuticals? Perhaps the best answer is that, before experimenting with exotic dietary supplement ingredients, it first makes sense to start out with the three dietary supplements that everyone should be taking: a multivitamin, vitamin D, and omega-3 fatty acids.

Multivitamin

The research above makes a good case for the daily use of a multivitamin as a nutrition insurance policy that helps to fill in the gaps for those nutrients people may not be getting in their diet. Furthermore, in a study of 90,771 men and women, the regular use of a multivitamin was found to significantly improve adequate intake of nutrients compared to nonusers. Also, recent research found that multivitamin supplements are generally well tolerated, do not increase the risk of mortality, cerebrovascular disease, or heart failure, and their use likely outweighs any risk in the general population (and may be particularly beneficial for older people).

So, the bottom line is that multivitamins really do work as a nutrition insurance policy.

Other Multivitamin Benefits

In addition to functioning as a nutrition insurance policy, the daily use of a multivitamin may offer other benefits as well.

Cardiovascular: A twelve-week, randomized, placebo-controlled study of 182 men and women (24 to 79 years) found that a multivitamin was able to lower homocysteine levels and the oxidation of LDL cholesterol—both of which are highly beneficial in reducing the risk for cardiovascular disease. Other multivitamin research has also demonstrated effectiveness in lowering homocysteine levels. A 6-month, randomized, double-blind, placebo-controlled study of 87 men and women (30 to 70 years) found that multivitamin use was associated with lower levels of C-reactive protein, a measurement of inflammation associated with cardiovascular disease and other degenerative diseases. Other multivitamin research in women has shown similar results.

Sweden

A Swedish population-based case-control study of 1,296 men and women (45 to 70 years) who previously had a heart attack and 1,685 healthy men and women as controls found that those using a multivitamin were less likely to have a heart attack. Other multivitamin research in Swedish women has shown similar results.

Cancer: A large-scale, randomized, double-blind, placebo-controlled study was conducted with 14,641 male US physicians initially 50 years or older, including 1,312 men with a history of cancer, to determine the long-term effects of multivitamin supplementation on incidence of various types of cancers. Results showed that during a median follow-up of 11.2 years, men with a history of cancer who took a daily multivitamin had a statistically significant reduction in the incidence of total cancer compared to those taking a placebo.

Stress/Energy: A human clinical study with 96 healthy men (18 to 46 years) examined the effect of multivitamin supplementation in relation to plasma interleukin-6 (IL-6, a proinflammatory chemical produced by the body) and anger, hostility, and severity of depressive symptoms. The results showed that plasma IL-6 was associated with anger, hostility, and severity of depressive symptoms, and that multivitamin use was associated with lower plasma IL-6 levels. Patients complaining of fatigue, tiredness, and low energy levels may have low levels of vitamins and minerals. Supplementation with nutrients including B vitamins (e.g., a multivitamin) can alleviate deficiencies, but supplements must be taken for an adequate period of time.

A meta-analysis of eight randomized and placebo-controlled studies evaluated the influence of diet supplementation on stress and mood. Results showed that supplementation reduced the levels of perceived stress, mild psychiatric symptoms, anxiety, fatigue, and confusion. Supplements containing high doses of B vitamins (e.g., multivitamins) may be more effective in improving mood states.

Aging: At the ends of our chromosomes are those stretches of DNA called telomeres that you've already heard so much about. These telomeres protect our genetic data, making it possible for cells to divide. Each time a cell divides, telomeres get shorter. When they get too short, the cell can no longer divide and becomes inactive or "senescent" or dies. This process is associated with aging. In a cross-sectional analysis of data from 586 women (35 to 74 years), multivitamin use was assessed, and relative telomere length was measured. The results were that multivitamin use was significantly associated with longer telomeres. Compared with nonusers, the relative telomere length was on average 5.1 percent longer among daily multivitamin users. It is possible, therefore, that multivitamins may help us live longer.

Each one of us should be taking the three key dietary supplements: a multivitamin, vitamin D, and omega-3 fatty acids.

Vitamin D

Vitamin D is the "sunshine vitamin," so coined because exposure to the sun's ultraviolet light will convert a form of cholesterol under the skin into vitamin D. This nutrient is best known for its role in helping to facilitate the absorption of calcium and phosphorus (as well as magnesium), thus helping to promote bone health. Over the past decade, however, research on vitamin D has identified numerous other roles it plays in human health and wellness, which include:

- Inhibiting the uncontrolled proliferation of cells (as in the case of cancer) and stimulating the differentiation of cells (specialization of cells for specific functions);
- Helping prevent cancers of the prostate and colon;
- Functioning as a potent immune system modulator;
- Helping prevent autoimmune reactions;
- Helping improve insulin secretion;
- Decreasing the risk of high blood pressure via the renin-angiotensin system's regulation of blood pressure;
- Reducing osteoporotic fractures;
- Reducing the incidence of falls in older adults;
- Reducing the risk of developing premenstrual syndrome (PMS);
- Reducing the prevalence of depression, especially in the elderly; and
- Reducing the prevalence of urinary infections and lower urinary tract symptoms (e.g., benign prostatic hyperplasia or BPH).

Vitamin D deficiency and insufficiency: Outright vitamin D deficiency is present in 41.6 percent of the US population, while vitamin D insufficiency (i.e., lacking sufficient vitamin D) is present in 77 percent of the population. If you are deficient in vitamin D, you will not be able to absorb enough calcium to satisfy your body's calcium needs. It has long been known that severe vitamin D deficiency has serious consequences for bone health, but other research indicates that lesser degrees of vitamin D deficiency are common and increase the risk of osteoporosis and other health problems.

Vitamin D sufficiency is measured by serum 25-hydroxyvitamin D levels in the body. Laboratory reference ranges for serum 25-hydroxyvitamin D levels are based upon average values from healthy populations. However, recent research examining the prevention of secondary hyperparathyroidism and bone loss suggest that the range for healthy 25-hydroxyvitamin D levels should be considerably higher.

Based upon the most current research, here are the ranges for serum 25-hydroxyvitamin D values:

- Less than 20–25 nmol/L: Indicates severe deficiency associated with rickets and osteomalacia;

- 50–80 nmol/L: Previously suggested as normal range; and

- 75–125 nmol/L: More recent research suggests that parathyroid hormone and calcium absorption are optimized at this level; this is a healthy range.

Based upon the 75–125 nmol/L range, it is estimated that one billion people in the world are currently vitamin D deficient. Furthermore, research indicates that supplementation with at least 800–1,000 IU daily are required to achieve serum 25-hydroxyvitamin D levels of at least 80 nmol/L. Furthermore, there are many groups of individuals who currently are at risk for vitamin D deficiency. These include:

- Exclusively breast-fed infants: Especially if they do not receive vitamin D supplementation and if they have dark skin and/or receive little sun exposure;

- Dark skin: People with dark-colored skin synthesize less vitamin D from sunlight than those with light-colored skin. In a US study, 42 percent of African American women were vitamin D deficient compared to 4 percent of white women;

- The elderly: When exposed to sunlight, the elderly have reduced capacity to synthesize vitamin D;

- Those using sunscreen: Applying sunscreen with an SPF factor of 8 reduces production of vitamin D by 95 percent;

- Those with fat malabsorption syndromes: The absorption of dietary vitamin D is reduced in cystic fibrosis and cholestatic liver disease;

- Those with inflammatory bowel disease: An increased risk of vitamin D deficiency occurs in those with inflammatory bowel disease like Crohn's disease; and

- Obese individuals: Obesity increases the risk of vitamin D deficiency.

Vitamin D2 and D3

There are two forms of vitamin D available as a dietary supplement: cholecalciferol (vitamin D3) and ergocalciferol (vitamin D2). Cholecalciferol is the form made in the human body, and it is more active than ergocalciferol. In fact, Vitamin D2 potency is less than one-third that of vitamin D3. Commercially, ergocalciferol is derived from yeast and so is considered vegetarian, while cholecalciferol is commonly derived from lanolin (from sheep) or fish oil—although a vegetarian D3 derived from lichen is available. Ideal dosing for vitamin D, according to the Linus Pauling Institute, is that generally healthy adults take 2,000 IU of supplemental vitamin D daily. The Vitamin D Council states that if well adults and adolescents regularly avoid sunlight exposure, then it is necessary to supplement with at least 5,000 IU of vitamin D daily. The Council for Responsible Nutrition recommends 2,000 IU daily for adults. Taking a conservative position, at least 2,000 IU of vitamin D makes sense for adults.

Omega-3 Fatty Acids

Chemically, a fatty acid is an organic acid that has an acid group at one end of its molecule and a methyl group at the other end. Fatty acids are typically categorized in the omega groups 3, 6, and 9 according to the location of their first double bond (there's also an omega 7 group, but these are less important to human health). The body uses fatty acids for the formation of healthy cell membranes, the proper development and functioning of the brain and nervous system, and for the production of hormone-like substances called eicosanoids (thromboxanes, leukotrienes, and prostaglandins). These chemicals regulate numerous body functions including blood pressure, blood viscosity, vasoconstriction, and immune and inflammatory responses.

Deficiency of Omega-3 Fatty Acids

While omega-3, -6, and -9 fatty acids are all important for different reasons, it is the omega-3 fatty acids (O3FA) that are currently particularly critical—and specifically the O3FA known as eicosapentaenoic acid (EPA) and docosahexaenoic acid (DHA). The reason for this current importance is that Western diets are deficient in O3FA and have excessive amounts of omega-6 fatty acids. While human beings evolved on a diet with approximately a 1:1 ratio of omega-6 to omega-3 fatty acids (EFA), the current Western diet provides about a 16:1 ratio. As a matter of fact, a recent Harvard School of Public Health study indicates that omega-3 deficiency causes 96,000 US deaths per year. Other research has clearly shown that excessive amounts of omega-6 fatty acids and a very high omega-6 to omega-3 ratio, as is found in today's Western diets, promote many diseases, including cardiovascular disease, cancer, and inflammatory and autoimmune diseases, whereas increased levels of omega-3 (a low omega-6 to omega-3 ratio) exert protective effects.

Benefits of Omega-3 Fatty Acids

O3FA offer a broad range of benefits in human health. These benefits are listed below categorically.

Cardiovascular: In several studies O3FA have been shown to help lower triglyceride levels. In fact, the FDA has even approved an O3FA product for this purpose. Individually, EPA and DHA also have triglyceride-lowering properties. Consuming 1 gram/day of fish oils from fish (about 3 ounces of fatty fish such as salmon) or fish oil supplements has a cardioprotective effect. Evidence suggests that increased consumption of O3FA from fish or fish-oil supplements, but not of alpha-linolenic acid, reduces the rates of all-cause mortality, cardiac and sudden death, and possibly stroke. Higher consumption of fish and O3FA has been associated with a lower risk of coronary heart disease. Clinical research shows that DHA supplementation helps increase HDL cholesterol levels (the "good cholesterol"). Supplementation with fish oil produces modest, but significant reductions in systolic and diastolic blood pressure in patients with mild hypertension.

Inflammation: O3FA have been shown to help relieve inflammation caused by a variety of factors.

Rheumatoid arthritis: Research has demonstrated that fish oil supplementation is effective in the treatment of rheumatoid arthritis.

Menopause: Clinical research shows that supplementing with 500 mg EPA, 3 times daily, modestly but significantly reduces the frequency of hot flashes compared to placebo in menopausal women.

ADHD: Research has shown children with attention deficit/hyperactive disorder (ADHD) may have low plasma levels of

EPA and DHA. Clinical research suggests that supplementation with DHA might improve aggression and social relationships in ADHD children.

Macular degeneration: Increased dietary consumption of DHA is associated with reducing the risk of macular degeneration.

Alzheimer's disease: Participants who consumed fish once per week or more had 60 percent less risk of Alzheimer disease compared with those who rarely or never ate fish, and this was attributed to the DHA content of the fish.

Do Omega-3 Fatty Acids Increase the Risk of Prostate Cancer?

According to a prospective study published in the *Journal of the National Cancer Institute* (JNCI), (1) a high intake of long-chain omega-3 fatty acids from foods and supplements could increase the risk of developing aggressive prostate cancer by 71 percent. So, does this mean that men should stop eating fish and supplementing with fish oil supplements? *No, it does not.* First, it should be noted that this JNCI study was a case–cohort study in which data was examined from a different study (The Selenium and Vitamin E Cancer Prevention Trial). This is significant because that means that this observational study was *not* designed to investigate the role of omega-3s in prostate cancer.

However, there have been other studies that were designed to do just that. A 2013 randomized, double-blind, placebo-controlled trial published in the *British Journal of Nutrition* (2) found that daily supplementation with EPA omega-3 fish oils significantly reduced prostate-specific antigen (PSA) levels, a measure of prostate cancer risk. In addition, a 2011 phase II prospective randomized trial published in *Cancer Prevention Research* (3) found that a low-fat diet with fish oil supplementation decreased prostate cancer proliferation. Another case-control study published in *Clinical Cancer Research* (4) found that dietary intake of omega-3 fatty acids was strongly associated with a decreased risk of aggressive prostate cancer.

The Sources of Omega-3 Fatty Acids

To begin with, the overwhelming majority of research on the health benefits of supplementation with O3FA has been conducted using fish oil products. Consequently, a strong argument can be made that fish oil supplements are the preferred source of O3FA. Amongst these, the primary fish used commercially as the source from which O3FA are derived include mackerel, herring, tuna, halibut, salmon, and cod liver. Although some fish are touted as superior over others as sources for supplemental fish oil, it is the opinion of this author that they all provide acceptable sources of omega-3s. Still, there are other sources of O3FA besides fish oil. This includes squid, krill, flax seed oil, and algae oil.

Squid: Squid-derived O3FA are derived from byproducts of squid that are usually discarded when squid are commercially fished and provides a much higher concentration of DHA (up to 50 percent) than does fish oil. However, there is a lack of human clinical data on squid-source O3FA, although they likely will have similar effects as fish oil.

Krill: Krill oil derived from the shrimp-like crustacean known as krill contain significant amounts of the EPA and DHA omega-3 fatty acids, as well as phospholipids (e.g., phosphatidylcholine), vitamin A, vitamin E, and astaxanthin, a powerful carotenoid antioxidant. Human clinical research has shown that krill oil has greater absorption than fish oil—although krill provides significantly less EPA/DHA per gram than fish oil.

Flax seed: Flax seed oil contains about 52–55 percent omega-3s, but as alpha-linolenic acid (ALA), not EPA/DHA. This is significant since ALA has to be converted to EPA and DHA before it will provide the much of touted health benefits attributed to O3FA. This is problematic since studies indicate that in men, approximately 8 percent of ALA is converted to EPA and 0–4 percent is converted to DHA. In women, approximately 21 percent of dietary ALA is converted to EPA and 9 percent is converted to DHA. This is not to say that flax seed oil has no value. It does, but just not as significant a value as fish oil.

Algae oil: Certain algae extracts provide a vegetarian source of O3FA, but in this case the O3FA are EPA and DHA, not ALA. Consequently, for vegetarians, algae oil is a viable substitute for fish oil. That being said, human clinical research on algae oil sources of O3FA is limited, and the cost is far more than fish oil.

Most of us are not getting all the nutrients we need from our diet. Consequently, we should all consider taking these three key dietary supplements to help compensate for these deficiencies: a *broad-spectrum multivitamin, vitamin D, and omega-3 fatty acids.* Not only will these supplements act as a nutritional insurance policy against inadequate nutrient intake, but each supplement also offers a range of health benefits associated with their regular use at optimal levels.

I take all three daily. For my broad-spectrum multivitamin, I take *Vitamere Ultra Anti Aging,* the most advanced multivitamin on the market that I developed in 2012. Not only does it have potent doses of all of the standard vitamins, minerals, and trace elements of a regular multivitamin, but it also has extra ingredients that help promote DNA health and telomere length. These ingredients were carefully researched and are supported by 402 scientific publications.

With the use of *Vitamere Ultra Anti Aging,* along with proper diet, exercise and healthy lifestyle habits, I was able to reverse biologic aging in my body, as measured by mean telomere length. Between 2012 and 2017, my biologic age went from that of thirty-nine year old to that of a twenty year old—not bad for someone sixty-two years of age. I am a good example of what can be achieved if we put our minds to it and make health a priority. Good health won't happen by accident for most people. They will have to be proactive and take control of their health.

CHAPTER 12

HEALTHY BLOOD VESSELS

How Important Are Your Blood Vessels?

They're critically important. Yet most people don't understand how they work until it's too late. Your body is full of blood vessels. They are your body's highways, boulevards, streets, and alleys. You can't see most of them other than the veins in your skin, but they are an excellent indicator of your overall health. You are only as healthy as your blood vessels. How you treat your blood vessels can determine how well you age. The vascular system is a magnificent and complex machine. The blood vessels of the circulatory system consist of:

1. Arteries: Blood vessels that carry oxygenated blood away from the heart to the body;

2. Veins: Blood vessels that carry blood from the body back into the heart; and

3. Capillaries: Tiny blood vessels between arteries and veins that distribute oxygen-rich blood to the body.

The good news is that the vascular system is relatively simple to understand. It is our body's plumbing system. Your vascular system distributes oxygen and nutrients throughout your body. The arteries carry oxygen and nutrients to the organs in your body while veins take away the waste matter back to the heart. The capillaries bridge the arteries and veins and allow the transfer of nutrients to the cells and tissues and carry away waste from them. Lymphatic vessels are special tubes that carry extracellular fluid and tissue fluid back to the heart outside of the venous system.

Without your blood vessels, your tissue and organs would not get oxygen and nutrients or eliminate waste. Partially clogged blood vessels reduce the efficiency of our organs, which can slow us down and make us sluggish. With a lack of circulation, we age faster. We need energy to function at our best. Without blood flow to supply us with the nutrients needed to produce energy, our system slows down and we become sluggish. With clogged pipes, you just can't do much.

Creating good health is a process of consistency and understanding. I'm not asking you to read this book and sign up for a 5k. What I am doing, however, is encouraging you to develop a routine of positive habits and changes that will impact your health today. You don't have to understand the human body like a neurosurgeon does. But you can educate yourself on the basics and give yourself the encouragement and momentum needed to make positive changes today!

How Your Blood Vessels Work

The inside of your arteries is composed of three layers. The innermost layer is called the tunica interna or intima. It is a simple epithelium surrounded by connective tissue. The middle layer is the tunica media, and it is primarily a smooth muscle layer and is usually the thickest layer of the three. The last layer is the tunica externa. It is composed of connective tissue made up of collagen.

Nitric oxide is a chemical compound produced by the endothelium cells, which line the blood vessel walls. It promotes vasodilation that lowers your blood pressure and prevents white blood cells from adhering to the artery walls. When white blood cells start adhering to the walls and plaque starts to gather, that is when you start seeing cardiovascular events. Nitric oxide also prevents platelet aggregation on the blood vessel wall, which prevents clot formation that can occlude an artery.

There's a layer between the blood plasma and endothelium called the glycocalyx. It is made of proteins called proteoglycans. The glycocalyx attaches to the endothelium cells themselves and determines what gets through to the endothelium. It manages the cells and nutrients that go through it. The glycocalyx protects the endothelial cells from cells that could cause clotting. Think of the glycocalyx as the offensive line protecting the quarterback. They modulate the inflammatory responses. They bind antioxidants and reduce oxidative stress. They also help capture free radicals and reduce the damage that they can cause to the endothelial cells and tissue.

Free radicals attach to nitric oxide, stealing the oxygen and making it unusable. You've heard about free radicals, which cause damage to cells, but may not really know much about them. Antioxidants are so important because they neutralize the free radicals so that they don't damage healthy tissue. The glycocalyx is your defense, but it can only protect you up to a certain point. If you overwhelm it with free radicals, you will destroy the glycocalyx. It won't be able to modulate the inflammatory response. The glycocalyx can be disrupted by a sugary meal. One bad high-carb meal can cause you to lose 50 percent of your glycocalyx. High cholesterol also diminishes the glycocalyx.

The glycocalyx is the first line of defense in your blood vessels between the blood and the blood vessel wall. The next line of defense is your endothelium. If they get past those defenses, then the blood vessels can become diseased and develop plaque, which can lead to cardiac problems and blood clots. Again, it all goes back to healthy eating, exercise, and developing healthy lifestyle habits.

When endothelium is unhealthy, it makes less nitric oxide. The less nitric oxide, the more your arteries are constricted and the less blood that flows through the artery. Endothelial cells are important, and when they are sick, they don't produce enough nitric oxide. This can cause platelets to start adhering to the blood vessel wall, potentially producing a blood clot, which puts you at risk for heart attack or stroke. If you've ever been around someone who has had a stroke, you can see how devastating that can be. So, keep your glycocalyx and your endothelium in tip-top shape so you can enjoy good health well into the future.

THE REASON WHY YOU NEED HEALTHY BLOOD VESSELS IS TO HAVE GOOD BLOOD FLOW SO THAT YOU CAN DELIVER MAXIMAL AMOUNTS OF OXYGEN AND NUTRIENTS TO YOUR ORGANS AND TISSUES.

Lifestyle habits can affect the rheology of blood, or how blood flows through blood vessels. The viscosity (how thick a fluid is) of blood can be impacted by poor lifestyle habits as you get older. As your blood gets thicker, it can start to cause problems. Viscosity can be increased by an increase in fibrinogen levels in the blood or by decreased red blood cell deformability.

Red blood cells have the ability to change shape to allow for better flow. It's called red blood cell deformability. If they lose that ability, they have trouble changing shape to move more efficiently through the arteries and capillaries. This is where the blood cells can start to stick to themselves. The reason this occurs with age is due to increased inflammation and oxidative stress from free radicals. Fibrinogen levels also rise because of these very same factors. This is a double whammy as far as blood viscosity is concerned.

Doctors and neurologists know this fact that I'm about to share with you, but most people have a hard time believing it. Google it or ask a medical expert such as a neurosurgeon if you need confirmation. You're about to see that the human body has a *lot* of blood vessels!

It has been estimated that an adult has about 100,000 miles of blood vessels if you were to take them out and lay them end to end. That means that your blood vessels would wrap around the earth 4 times. That many miles of blood vessels shows you just how important they are. Most people take their blood vessels for granted and don't take preventative measures to ensure their health. After all, they can't see or feel them, so how can they know that anything is wrong? In many cases, they don't find out until it is too late. Fifty percent of first heart attacks present as sudden death. By then it is too late. The other 50 percent at that point usually start paying attention. But by then, damage has been done.

The time to start paying attention to your blood vessels is right now.

The time to start paying attention to your blood vessels is right now. The state of their health will determine your longevity and level of function. What if you could use the knowledge you gain here to make positive changes that increase your blood vessel health?

Usually Your Arteries Begin to Close Off Very Slowly

It begins with inflammation occurring in the lining of your arteries, in the intimal layer. It can then progress to deposition of fatty cholesterol and triglyceride molecules in the blood vessel wall itself, producing plaque. As the plaque grows, the blood vessel lumen begins to get smaller and smaller, allowing less and less blood to get through. Eventually the blood vessel can become completely clogged and all blood flow stops, at which point the organ or tissue that it supplies dies if no collateral blood flow has developed by then. Sometimes even a small plaque that is hemodynamically insignificant can rupture, causing the blood in that artery to clot, completely clogging the artery before any collateral blood flow develops, resulting in a sudden catastrophic event such as a major heart attack or massive stroke.

We now have testing that can look at the health of your arteries in a noninvasive way. It is a test known as the Carotid Artery IMT Scan. It uses ultrasound to image your carotid arteries in your neck. These are the arteries that go to your brain. It enables us to see if your intimal layer is thickened and whether or not you have plaque developing in the carotid artery wall. We can even tell if your artery is beginning to close off. If this study is abnormal, then you potentially could be sitting on a time bomb, and it is time to pay serious attention to your health.

YOUR BODY IS A VERY COMPLICATED MACHINE. ALL THE PIECES WORK TOGETHER. YOU HAVE TO TAKE CARE OF ALL THE PARTS.

High cholesterol, inflammation, and high blood pressure are very detrimental to your blood vessel health. They are silent killers. They initially cause no symptoms, so you don't think anything is wrong, but they are quietly working behind the scenes, causing damage to your blood vessels and, as a result, your body. The good news is we have ways to detect abnormal levels of cholesterol, blood pressure, and inflammation. But if you don't look, you will never find it. The key is to be proactive and find the problem in its infancy before it becomes a clinical problem.

Often, I encounter people who believe that their health issues happen by accident or are a fault of their genetics. They seem surprised when they have a cardiovascular event. But when I ask them about their lifestyle habits, it turns out they have not worked out consistently or eaten the right foods. Then there are the people who go to the gym on a regular basis but never see a change in their body composition, as they are never able get a handle on their diet.

They are consistently eating high-glycemic, low-nutritional value, processed foods full of high glycemic carbohydrates, sugar, salt, and fat. Why do people sabotage their health? There are many reasons including lack of knowledge as well as lack of self-control and discipline. But it's you who must take the initiative. You control your health by how you live your live. What do you want your level of function to be now and in the future?

DOCTORS DON'T CURE ANYTHING; WE HELP THE BODY HEAL ITSELF. WE DON'T HEAL ANYTHING; WE JUST HELP THE BODY DO ITS JOB.

When you study down to the cellular level, you can really see the difference that lifestyle makes. If you get enough nutrients and oxygen to your cells and organs, they will heal themselves. When the damage in your body exceeds your natural repair mechanisms, that's when you get old.

Why Do People Get Sick?

The basic answer for most is an unhealthy lifestyle. I get sick maybe once a year. Yet in all my years as a neurosurgeon and practicing as an age-management doctor, I have never taken a sick day. I have never gotten sick enough to miss work! Ever. I deal with sick people all day long, so you'd think I would get sick, too, but I've never missed a day of work in thirty-seven years due to illness. When you are healthy, you fight off infection and disease. You need good health to have a good immune system. To have good health, you have to practice healthy lifestyle habits.

If your immune system doesn't work, then even antibiotics won't help. You have to make your health a priority every day.

CHAPTER 13

SIMPLE NUTRITION

Are You Making Your Food More Complicated Than It Needs to Be?

Nutrition wasn't meant to be complicated. If you think about food and how it comes from its natural source, it is very simple. With the invention of "fast food" and restaurant dining, there is no real way to know what you are eating. Many additives that go into food are meant to make you think it tastes better. Sugar, salt, fat, preservatives, and MSG are all things that go into food as well as chemical additives that hide in labels under the name "natural flavors."

To truly be responsible for what you eat, you have to take it back to the way food was meant to be consumed—the simpler the better. The closer the food is to the way it comes out of the ground or grows on the bush or on tree, the better. If it swims, flies, or runs free range, you can eat it. The more food is changed from its original natural form and becomes processed, the worse it is for you.

A lot of today's foods don't look anything close to how they started. They have been changed, processed, and refined to make them look and taste irresistible. Sugar, salt, and fat in various forms as well as preservatives and artificial flavors are the most common additives and are ubiquitous in most of our foods. Specialty food companies can manufacture chemical flavors that make food taste any way you want it. You name the taste, and they can compound a chemical to make it taste that way.

They then call it an "artificial flavor," but it is really a chemical. How that chemical impacts your health is anyone's guess, but from seeing a decline in the overall health of our population over the last forty years, you can bet it isn't a good impact.

Eat whole natural foods, foods that are real, preferably organic and free range, so as not be exposed to chemicals, antibiotics, pesticides, and toxins. Eat nutrient-dense but calorie-light foods, such as vegetables. You can eat all the green leafy vegetables you want. They will fill you up with comparably few calories. Minimize calorie dense foods such as starchy root vegetables.

Stay away from sugar and refined carbohydrates. They will spike your sugar and insulin, making it impossible to burn fat for fuel. You will instead constantly store fat, especially around your belly. Remember that belly fat creates estrogen, and that can result in hormone imbalances. Everything is connected.

STAY AWAY FROM TROPICAL FRUIT SUCH AS BANANAS, PINEAPPLE, KIWI, MANGO, PAPAYA, MELON, CANTALOUPE, AND WATERMELON. THEY ALL HAVE TOO MUCH SUGAR.

Eat lots of lean protein such as fish, chicken, turkey, pork tenderloin (sorry, Rabbi), bison, ostrich (one of my favorites), egg whites, beans, lentils, and fat-free or low-fat cottage cheese if no dairy allergies.

Apples, pears, and oranges are okay but not fruit juices as fruit juice is just concentrated sugar without the fiber and pulp to slow down the absorption of sugar. Sugar too easily becomes an addiction for the human body. It is *your Trojan horse.* It tastes and feels good going down, but then it destroys you from within.

Berries are your best bet as they have reasonable amounts of sugar and don't spike your blood sugar too badly. Strawberries have the least amount of sugar of most berries, followed by black-berries, blueberries, and raspberries. Portion control is important with fruit as you can overload your body with sugar if you eat too much. The order that you consume your food is important, too. Always eat some protein or a healthy fat before or with fruit to decrease the blood sugar spike. I often eat nuts or some Jarlsberg cheese or even avocado when eating fruit. It is also a good idea to do this if you are drinking wine, as wine is full of sugar.

When Eating Carbohydrates, Some Rules Apply

Avoid all high glycemic carbohydrates. This includes sweets, pro-cessed carbohydrates, starchy vegetables, and tropical and dried fruits. The more you eat, the more you crave. Avoid them, and the cravings will go away. Never eat a carbohydrate by itself!

Always balance with protein and good fats; an example is an apple with a handful of raw, unsalted nuts.

Never eat a carbohydrate by itself!

Evening meals and snacks *must* be low glycemic. Insulin and growth hormone are com-petitors for the same IGF1 receptor, so if insulin is around, growth hormone won't be able to do its job. Growth hormone is released during sleep. If insulin levels are high, growth hormone cannot access cells as the receptors on the cells will be bound to insulin molecules, and your body will not get the benefits of growth hor-mone, which is responsible for repair and rejuvenation of tissue.

Pick your poison carefully, and restrict your intake of high-glycemic carbs as much as possible. Even when balanced with a protein or a good fat, high-glycemic carbohydrates are best *after* exercise. Adrenaline, which is released during exercise, remains active for about one-hour post-exercise and suppresses insulin. This creates a one-hour time frame when carbohydrates can be readily absorbed to replenish muscle glycogen.

Enjoy a Free Day Once a Week

Eat for your health and energy six days a week, and on your free day, eat for everything else (social events, emotional needs, preferences, etc.). Cheating a little every day will increase insulin levels on a chronic basis, while having "bad foods" just once a week in moderation will not. By restricting high-glycemic carbs to just one day a week, you have six days of low insulin levels and just one of higher levels. On balance, you win. If you cheat every day, your insulin levels remain high seven days a week, and you lose.

Back to Nature

The eating plan we recommend in our age-management practice is most reminiscent of the Paleolithic nutrition eaten by our ancestors. They ate nutrient-dense foods such as fruits, vegetables, lean meats, essential fats, and virtually no refined or overly processed fats or simple carbohydrates. For thousands of years, humans ate very simply: if it grew from the ground, fell from the trees, swam or ran across our path, we ate it.

Since it took thousands of years for our digestive systems to adapt to the addition of small amounts of grains and dairy products, there is no way our bodies could have adapted to the additives, preservatives, colorings, and flavorings that now dominate our food choices. Even natural products like sugar have taken a very unnatural turn.

Government research shows that in 1999, sugar consumption per person averaged 158 pounds per year! That is a far cry from our sugar-free hunter/gatherer days. Our bodies have not had a chance to catch up with the dietary changes we have made, and the results have been disastrous. The rates of heart attacks, type II diabetes, obesity, strokes, hypertension, and gastrointestinal disorders in this country just keep climbing. Fortunately, all of these conditions can be greatly improved by positive dietary changes.

Omega-3 Eggs

Omega-3 eggs are laid by chickens that have been fed flaxseeds. The eggs actually contain more omega-3 fatty acids, a healthy essential fat, and less saturated fat than those laid by grain/corn-fed chickens.

Free Range/Organic/Grass-Fed

- Organic refers to the lack of chemicals present in the growing of a plant or raising of an animal.

- Free-range animals eat grass. Their meats contain a better ratio of good to bad fats compared to traditionally raised animals that are kept in small pens and fed grains to fatten them up faster. Grass contains omega-3 fatty acids which have anti-inflammatory effects, whereas grains contain more omega-6 fatty acids, which have a pro-inflammatory effect.

- Nonorganic meats contain certain amounts of antibiotics and bovine growth hormone. Hormone-free animal foods and dairy are recommended if you have access to them and can spare the greater expense.

- Nonorganic fruits and vegetables may contain pesticides and chemicals. Always wash your fruits and vegetables thoroughly.

Processed Foods, in Their Most Natural Form

- When choosing a packaged food, choose those that are minimally processed with the most natural ingredients.

- Whole grains are always the best option.

- Natural peanut butter is a great source of essential fatty acids, while processed peanut butter is a source of sugar and hydrogenated oil.

- Whole/ground flax seeds are a source of omega-3 fatty acid, while flaxseed oil is directly linked to prostate cancer in men.

- Farm-raised fish, labeled "Atlantic," have lower essential fatty acid content then their "wild"/"ocean" fish counterparts. They are also lower in protein and higher in saturated fat. Most "Atlantic" fish have added food coloring.

- Fat-free dairy products are usually supplemented with sugar to make them palatable, so be aware and read the label.

- Instant rice and instant oatmeal have a higher glycemic index than their slow-cooking counterparts because the surrounding husk has been removed.

I like to always know how food impacts my blood sugar, so I measure it whenever I introduce new food to my diet that may be glycemic. Here are some sample blood sugar measurements I did on myself, using a glucometer, to see the impact of a food or meal on my blood sugar. I tested my blood sugar at baseline (before eating), then 30, 60, 90, and occasionally 120 minutes after the meal. Once my blood sugar dropped below one hundred, I usually stopped measuring, so not all examples go out to the 120-minute mark.

My goal is to not eat a food or a meal if it spikes my blood sugar above 110–120 thirty to sixty minutes following ingestion.

Meal: Gala apple
Baseline: 94

30 min: 131
60 min: 107
90 min: 94

Note the spike in my blood sugar to 131 at the 30-minute mark.
I then ate some protein and fat prior to eating the apple and here
are the results:

Meal: 2 oz. mixed nut, 1 oz. Jarlsberg cheese, then a gala apple
Baseline: 85
30 min: 102
60 min: 85
90 min: ND

Note the dramatic attenuation of my blood sugar from 131 at
the 30-minute mark to 102. Never eat a carb without a protein or
fat before it.

Here is another example:

Meal: 1 can black beans
Baseline: 77
30 min: 119
60 min: 103
90 min: 90

On a different day, I then ate one avocado with the black beans
at the same time. Here are the results:

Meal: 1 can black beans and 1 avocado

Baseline: 78
30 min: 89
60 min: 86

Once again, we see the 30-minute sugar level dropping from 119 to 89 and the 60-minute blood sugar dropping from 103 to 86.

Here is an example of a high-glycemic fruit: cherries.

Meal: 11 Cherries
Baseline: 86
30 min: 158
After 50 min of cardio: 70

I was surprised to see my blood sugar spike to 158 at the 30-minute mark. I then got on my elliptical and did 50 minutes of cardio, and my blood sugar dropped to 70. So, if you are going to eat high glycemic fruit or carbs, do it right before an intense cardio workout so you can burn it off quickly. Cardio works well to reduce blood sugar. Your muscles burn it for fuel.

Here I ate some cheese right before eating the same amount of cherries.

Meal: 2.33 oz Jarlsberg cheese, 11 cherries
Baseline: 87
30 min: 117
60 min: 89

Note the addition of cheese with the cherries attenuated the spike in blood sugar at the 30-minute mark from 158 to 117.

Here is another example of protein attenuating the sugar spike:

Meal: 6 oz. blueberries from Texas
Baseline 94
30 min: 106
60 min: 104
90 min: 96

Meal: 6 oz. Texas blueberries, 16 oz. fat-free cottage cheese
Baseline: 75
30 min: 95
60 min: 85
90 min: ND

Note the attenuation of sugar at the 30-minute mark from 106 to 95 and at the 60-minute mark from 104 to 85.

Here is an example, which on the surface looked like a low-glycemic meal but really wasn't:

Meal: BBQ ribs, baked beans, cole slaw
Baseline: 81
30 min: 119
60 min: 123
90 min: 95

In this example, my blood sugar spiked more than I had expected. The reason why is that the barbecue sauce had a lot of sugar in it. The next day, I repeated this meal but wiped off as much of the barbecue sauce as I could. Here are the results:

Meal: BBQ ribs with sauce wiped off, baked beans with sauce washed off, cole slaw
Baseline: 88
30 min: 110
60 min: 102
90 min: 95

You can see the big improvement with the 30-minute blood sugar going from 119 to 110 and the 60-minute blood sugar going from 123 to 102.

Here are some values for berries, my favorite go-to fruit:

Strawberries:

Meal: 6 oz. strawberries
Baseline: 86
30 min: 109
60 min: 94
90 min: ND

Blackberries:

Meal: 6 oz. blackberries
Baseline: 82
30 min: 111
60 min: 101
90 min: 84

Blueberries from Mexico:

Baseline: 84
30 min: 123
60 min: 109
90 min: 92

Blueberries from Texas (it was early in the season and they were not as sweet as the blueberries from Mexico):

Meal: 6 oz. blueberries from Texas
Baseline 94
30 min: 106
60 min: 104

90 min: 96

Here are some examples of low glycemic meals:

Meal: sweet potato fries, tomato, flank steak
Baseline: 82
30 min: 102
60 min: 93
90 min: ND

Meal: salad, 1 can sardines
Baseline: 82
30 min: 94
60 min: 91
90 min: ND

Meal: large salad, 2 chicken breasts
Baseline: 82
30 min: 98
60 min: 88

Meal: large salad, 1 chicken breast, 6 oz. tuna fish
Baseline: 84
30 min: 90
60 min: 84

Here is a comparison of Quaker Oats steel-cut slow-cooked oatmeal and One Minute Quaker Oats oatmeal, which are rolled very thin to expose the endosperm so it cooks faster. The one-minute oatmeal is ready in one minute. The steel-cut oatmeal cooks for thirty minutes. The endosperm is the portion of the seed/ grain that holds the carbs. The bran is the outer portion of the grain, and the germ is the embryo inside the grain that could potentially develop into a new plant. The endosperm provides energy for the seed.

Meal: Quaker Oats steel-cut slow-cooked whole grain oatmeal
Baseline: 83
30 min: 89
60 min: 84
90 min: 91
120 min: 73

Meal: Quaker Oats 1-minute rolled oats
Baseline: 86
30 min: 104
60 min: 104
90 min: 94

Note that at all time points, blood sugar levels are significantly higher for the quick, one-minute rolled oats as compared to the slow-cooked, steel-cut oats. Steel cut oats are the healthier choice.

Everyone's body is different, but they all work by the same rules and principles. The physiology is the same. If something is going to spike my blood sugar, it is going to spike yours, too.

When you eat poorly, you create inflammation in the body, which will lead to chronic disease including arthritis. Arthritis is preventable. Rather than treating the symptoms with medications, treat the root cause by adopting healthy lifestyle habits. When it comes to lifestyle change, a lot of times there is strength in numbers. People think we have to age. Everyone gets old, but not everyone has to age.

MOST PEOPLE ARE NOT GETTING ALL THE NUTRIENTS THEY NEED FROM THEIR DIET.

How do you stick to your lifestyle change, your age-management program, when your loved ones don't? This can be a challenge. Someone is more likely to listen to a doctor than a spouse. Part of changing a lifestyle that is not healthy is showing that person what their lifestyle is doing to their health and their body. When you go through the testing we talked about in this book and you see what you are doing to yourself, it can give you the motivation to change for the better. Inaction is not an option. Sticking your head in the sand won't work. You will get overwhelmed with chronic diseases and illness.

When you find yourself up against a spouse or loved one that won't be supportive and doesn't want to change, do what you need to do to stay healthy. Buy your own food and prepare it if necessary. If they want to

When you find yourself up against a spouse or loved one that won't be supportive and doesn't want to change, do what you need to do to stay healthy.

continue eating junk, don't be a facilitator. Make them shop for it themselves. There is no reason for you to have two standards. What is healthy for you is also healthy for your spouse. Good habits are just that: good habits.

Don't be an enabler. If you have people in your life who won't make the healthy choices, don't be the person who brings home donuts. For high-energy people who want to accomplish things in life, energy is everything. If you don't have energy, then you are going to struggle. Without proper lifestyle habits, your energy levels will be low.

It is debatable whether we should eat grains at all. There are so many vegetables to choose from, so why would you need to eat grains? There are so many lean proteins, too: ostrich, bison, seafood, chicken, turkey, legumes, and black beans to mention a few. Throw in some avocado for a healthy fat to slow down the sugar spike.

Sugar is poison to your system. You should eat as many non-starchy vegetables as you can get your hands on. They are calorie light and nutrient rich. You can't overeat them. Use olive oil as a salad dressing. Eat as much lean protein as it takes to keep you full 3–4 hours. If you are hungry before then, you are not eating enough protein. If you are not hungry in four hours, cut down the amount.

FOOD CAN BE MEDICINE, OR FOOD CAN BE POISON. YOU DETERMINE WHICH IT IS BY WHAT YOU PUT IN YOUR MOUTH. IF YOU EAT THE WRONG FOODS, IT WILL MAKE YOU OLD AND SICK FAST.

Eat only complex naturally occurring carbs: vegetables, fruit, whole grains, beans, nuts, quinoa, and steel-cut oats. Never eat processed carbs: bread, pasta, cupcakes, cereal, pizza, pastries, cookies, and so on. If eating carbs, always have some protein or a healthy fat before the carb. It will slow the absorption of sugar.

Avoid tropical fruit and fruit high in sugar, such as banana, pineapple, mango, cantaloupe, melon, and watermelon. I usually eat an apple, pear, or orange before doing cardio. It provides a good boost of energy for the workout, and the sugar burns off fast. Serving sizes are something we need to constantly be aware of. It is the art of not overeating. Think about food the proper way—as a fuel for your mind, body, and soul.

Examples of serving sizes can include:

Grains: 1/2 cup quinoa or brown rice

Vegetables: 1 cup equivalent of vegetables is 1 cup raw vegetable or vegetable juice; 2 cups leafy salad greens

Fruits: 1 cup equivalent is 1 cup fruit

Protein foods (meat, poultry, fish, dry beans, and nuts): 1 oz. equivalent is 1 oz. lean meat, poultry, or seafood; 2 egg whites or 1 egg; 1/4 cup cooked beans; 1 Tbsp. peanut butter; 1/2 oz. unsalted nuts/seeds. Note that 1/4 cup cooked beans equals 1 oz. protein equivalent, but 1/2 cup cooked beans equals 1 vegetable.

Dairy foods (Milk, Yogurt, and Cheese): 1 cup equivalent is 1 cup milk or yogurt; 1 1/2 oz. natural cheese, such as cheddar cheese; or 2 oz. processed cheese

Another way to think of it:

One cup of raw leafy vegetables or a sweet potato should be about the size of a small fist.

Three ounces of cooked lean meat or poultry is about the size of a deck of cards.

A teaspoon of soft margarine is about the size of one die.

You're the difference maker. The difference in how well you age is you.

An ounce and a half of fat-free or low-fat cheese is about the size of four stacked dice.

What's Next?

You're the difference maker. The difference in how well you age is you. No one else is better at getting it done. The more consistent you are, the more energy you will have, and energy is everything! I've given you a lot of information but now the rest of the journey is up to you. Don't forget the basics.

- Eat right; make healthy food choices. Eat real food; don't eat junk.

- Exercise regularly, preferably six days a week.

- Incorporate aerobic high-intensity exercise into your routine as well as weight training.

- Start a sensible nutritional supplementation regimen to fill in the gaps left by an imperfect diet in an imperfect world. A good starting point is a broad spectrum multivitamin, such as *Vitamere Anti Aging* or *Vitamere Ultra Anti Aging* as well as vitamin D and fish oil.

- Get your blood work done! It's important to know what is going on inside your body. Are your biomarkers of health and hormones at levels where they need to be? Are they at optimal levels? Are you in optimal health?

There is no better time to start then right now, so get to work! Your future is waiting for you.

PATIENT TESTIMONIALS

A few words from people who have made radical and positive changes to their health:

"I had seen his ads, and the fact that he was a neurosurgeon was really interesting to me. Then, my mom showed me his ad and said, "This was one of your dad's residents." Now I was definitely interested. My dad was chief of neurosurgery at UT Southwestern and Dr. Rosenstein was one of his chief residents.

Even so, even before I met him, I had a lot of trust in him since he had been trained by my father.

I was already working on my health, but I wasn't getting the results I wanted. When I went to see Dr. R., he evaluated me and changed the way I was doing things. He switched me to a low-glycemic diet, increased the amount of cardio I was doing, and changed the supplements I was taking.

When I got to the end of the quarter, I knew there were various tests coming, so I followed his program to the letter. That way, if something was off on those tests, we would know that if

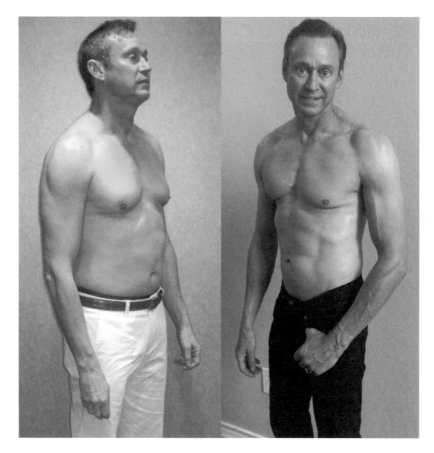

something was not right, it wasn't because I did not do the work. The tests helped make me accountable and gave me goals. And I improved each time.

Dr. Jacob Rosenstein's system is the best way to manage your health and wellness. He really understands the body's processes and the interactions. He goes beyond the numbers and works with the person, giving each patient a tailored plan to develop their own best health and longevity."

Peter Kemp Clark
Hager Oil and Gas Managing Partner

"I discovered Dr. Rosenstein several years ago, and his age-intervention program has had a dramatically positive impact on my health and wellbeing.

My body fat percentage has gone from the very high twenties to the very low teens. Weight has never been an issue until I learned how much of my weight was fat versus muscle. Those numbers are now in the right relationship with each other. That has resulted in a lower overall weight accompanied by five inches less waist diameter, better posture, and significant increase in strength plus muscle mass.

I sleep better and have energy far beyond my contemporaries.

I am currently six months past seventy-two and routinely work twelve-hour days with energy to spare. I found the right formula of diet, exercise, and nutritional supplements, following Dr. Rosenstein's plan and being inspired by his example.

This all might sound trite to you, but I assure you it is real. Dr. Rosenstein has an incredible personal and professional story. I consider him a friend as well as my health guide and doctor.

I recently asked him what the most rewarding aspect of his four-decade medical career was. His response? "Improving lives," which is a typical Jacob Rosenstein response—to the point and accurate. He surely has improved mine."

Mike Ames
Entrepreneur

"It has been a life-changing experience. Friends recommended that I see Dr. J, and it has given me new energy and new purpose. It helps us concentrate and focus on our health and well being. I have been married for thirty years, and our marriage is better than ever. And part of that is because of this program. I am seventy-one, and people ask me all the time when I am going to retire. I feel too young to retire!

My wife and I are in this together and it has become our hobby. Eating well and exercising together. We are enjoying life so much more than many of our friends that are our age."

Bill Rosenberry
Attorney

"Dr. Jacob's program has been life changing. I am sixty-four years old and I feel better than I did in my forties. I started this program while I was suffering through menopausal symptoms and it changed my experience moving through that aging stage as well as I have renewed energy and life. The program is life changing."

Donna Rosenberry

"My husband and I have been married for fifty years and that is a long time. When we decided to go through Dr Rosenstein's program we had both hit an age where we were really thinking about how we could best improve our health and our life to be the best we could be. The program revitalized our marriage. Our relationship has never been better and even in our near-seventies we have an active and healthy sex life! We have been in the program for ten years and through the program I have learned what I need to be doing in my life to stay healthy and active.

The earlier you can start Dr. Rosenstein's program the better off you will be for the rest of your life."

Sharon Walton

"Dr. Jacob's program made me healthier and happier of course. But the real way that it changed my life was the way it changed my wife and our relationship together. When we started the program, our marriage was suffering. Now this program has put our marriage at its best and we are both happier and healthier than we have ever been.

This program has been like turning back the clock at least ten years in so many ways. I am sixty-nine, and I plan to practice law and help my clients until I am at least eighty. I have no plans on retiring anytime soon, and that is different than many of my friends. I know that part of that is because of Dr. Rosenstein's program."

Rocky Walton
Attorney

"Dr. Rosenstein is one of the most brilliant doctors I have ever met. He is a perfectionist at all he does. He practices what he preaches, and he isn't a doctor that just tells you what to do to be successful, he does it and sees the results himself.

His age-management program has really helped me with this transition into the middle part of my life. It has helped me main-tain my energy and my athleticism. It has kept my body intact so that I can continue doing the things that I love to do. I know that being part of his program and taking his vitamins and supple-ments is what helped me heal from the life-changing back surgery he performed on me when I broke my back after being thrown off a horse. I don't know where I would be without him. I trust everything that he says. He walks the walk and talks the talk and lives it every day."

Jennifer Patterson
Attorney

"Dr. Rosenstein has always had a lot of credibility with me. He was my back surgeon. He is known in DFW as the doctor's doc-tor. I didn't know about age management before I met Dr. R. His program is incredible and has given me the energy and vitality to keep living a great life and being truly healthy. Unlike many doctors, who give you orders and ask you to follow them, Dr.

Rosenstein leads by example. He doesn't ask you to do anything that he wouldn't do himself. He says, 'Here is the road map. Here is what I do, and if you do this you will see change in your life.' I am grateful for his program and I hope to be in his age management program forever."

Mike Patterson
Attorney

"Like many professionals, I had come to the point where I was devoting my day to working in a sedentary position most of the day, as time slipped away. At age 60, I was 5'8', and 225 pounds and I was taking naps at 3 p.m. because I had no energy. My work efficiency dwindled. I had known Dr. R for many years, and he suggested I take a look at my biological health and life expectancy. My results shocked me because they showed that at age 60 I was the same as many Americans: overweight, with less libido and little time except for work, sleeping, and eating. That is what being successful in American business has to offer as a byproduct for many.

I am proud to be Dr. R's first patient. The before picture is a person I do not know. Today at age 70, I have vitality, endless energy, acute concentration, a more successful professional practice and time to enjoy what I worked so hard for: time with my family, children, and grandchildren.

My first test proved me to be borderline diabetic, and I had been diagnosed with early onset Parkinson's. I walked into Dr. R's office for a visit 4 months after starting the program and he was elated at my improvement and called his associates to visit. I went from 225 pounds to 165 pounds, and after 10 years I am still at 165. The blood tests proved each quarter how much I was improving. My Parkinson's has not progressed, and I no longer take Requip, which has side effects. My relationship with my wife and family has improved. At age 60 I was taking Effexor because of frustration; no longer! Please take a look at my before picture and my current picture ten years later. I don't know who that person in the before photo was!

Living in Europe for half of the year is even more telling. My friends ask if I have had plastic surgery as they see greater vitality and they say I look younger then they remember. The most gratifying experience is that I see a bright, positive, and enjoyable future for my life with my family, children, grandchildren, and by the way, my practice has doubled to what it was 10 years ago."

John A. Vann, PhD

"I know that Dr. Rosenstein's program truly does work, but it took a while for me to realize that it only works if you follow his instructions. For the past few years, I would swing between the Rosenstein program and the "doing what I wanted" way. Often after the results of my regular blood work would come in, I would sit down with Dr. Rosenstein to go over the numbers. My numbers weren't great in critical areas—mainly due to my choices—and I knew that he knew I was not following his plan for better nutrition and exercise as he had spelled out for me.

I just couldn't see how anyone could give up the good stuff (cookies, pizza, hamburgers, etc.) and be satisfied with veggies, fresh fruit, fish, nuts and supplements. One day shortly after a visit to his office, I decided to get serious and start following Dr. Rosenstein's program to the letter and change my bad habits to his plan for a healthy and more satisfying life. I cleared the house of all the "bad stuff" and started shopping to replace those things with the food choices he recommended. Next came exercise: six days a week of stretching and stationary bike.

I have been at my new lifestyle now for several months and things have certainly changed for me, just as Dr. Rosenstein said would happen. I no longer have cravings for sugary treats and carbs and I don't miss them at all, I look forward to meals of fresh vegetables, fruit, nuts, and lean meat. I take my supplements as directed, and the exercise that I dreaded now has become my time for planning my day and reflecting on what I've experienced. My hair and fingernails are both stronger and much healthier, my energy level is through the roof, I sleep like a baby, I love getting up to start my day and to top things off…I've lost twenty-five pounds. I am seventy-one years old and a true believer in his program!"

Joy Ames
Arlington, TX

"Dr. Rosenstein is the most impressive healthcare expert I've ever met in two decades. This is a book that won't just change your mindset. This is a book that could change your life."

Tammy Kling
CEO, OnFire Books Leadership Company

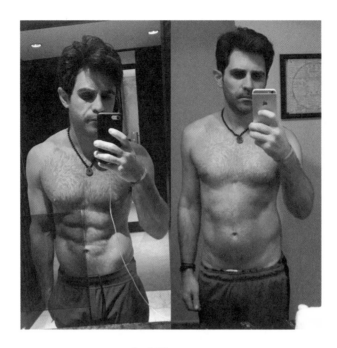

Ari Rastegar

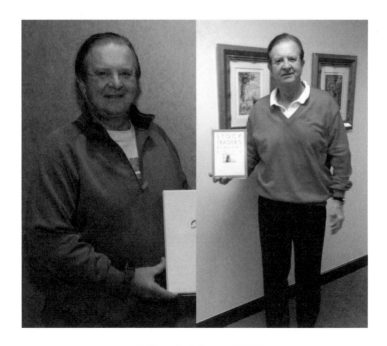

John A. Vann PhD

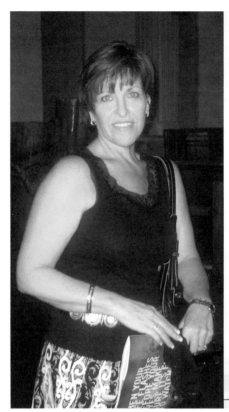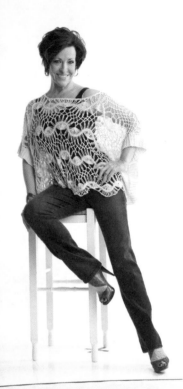

Judy Van Beest

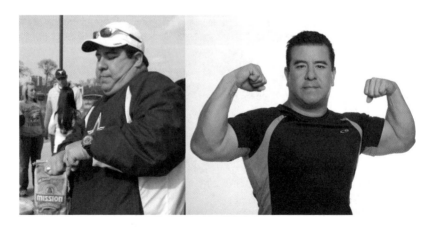

Mike Holguin

TIPS FOR STAYING MOTIVATED

- Keep a workout log to hold yourself accountable.

- Remember that you can live younger, feel younger, and be younger! Age is just a number.

- Remember why you are exercising (whether it is to lose weight, gain muscle, or have more energy).

- Change up your routine every two months. (Go for a run outdoors or take up hiking.)

- Work out with a partner if you can! But if not remember that in the end your health is up to you!

- Put your workout on your to-do list, and schedule time for it on your planner.

- Identify the excuses you like to use, and have a ready-made response.

- Remember that it is possible to reverse your age, by following this program in order to feel and look younger, have more vitality, and move more efficiently! How committed are you? How bad do you want it?

- Set short- and long-term goals to maximize success.

- Reward yourself for progress. Think outside of the edible rewards, such as new workout shoes or gear, new clothes, or a trip to the spa.

RULES FOR HEALTHY LIVING!

1. Before putting food in your mouth, ask yourself, "Will this food hurt me or heal me?"

2. Cherish your health, cherish your life.

3. Diets are a cover for poor lifestyle habits.

4. Adopt healthy habits. Don't just put lipstick on your bad ones.

5. Think positive thoughts and you will be happy. Think about misery and you'll get it!

6. Genetics loads the gun but environment pulls the trigger. Keep the safety on by making the right choices.

7. Food can turn your genes on and off. Good foods turn on your good genes and turn off the bad ones. What do you think bad foods do?

8. When you're healthy you perform better! Whether it's in the home, in the boardroom, or the bedroom.

9. The only thing they can't make more of is time. Once it's gone, it's gone. Time is priceless and cannot be replaced. Only you have the power to extend your timeline. You can determine how long or short it is by the choices you make in life.

10. Good health doesn't happen by accident. You have to pay attention.

11. Good health requires a desire to be and stay healthy and the knowledge of what it takes to get there and a plan to keep you there (desire, knowledge, execution, and staying power).

12. Good health is not a one-time event. It is a lifetime habit!

13. Sugar addiction is just as much a problem as opioid addiction. Opioids kill quickly while sugar takes its time.

14. You become what you think about.

15. You can't always believe what you see. A mirror may lie, but a picture tells the truth.

16. Fat and protein make you full. Sugar makes you hungry.

17. If you go through life oblivious to what it takes to be and stay healthy, you will sabotage your health-span, shorten your lifespan, and lengthen your "sick-span" or worse.

18. Food can be medicine or food can be poison. Be careful what you put in your mouth.

19. In an imperfect world with imperfect diets, nutritional supplements are essential to maintain your edge and lead a vital and vigorous life.

20. You control your health by how you live your life.

21. Imagine what you could do with the wisdom of the ages and the boundless energy and passion of youth!

TAKE CARE OF YOUR BRAIN HEALTH

Here are some immediate things you can do to prevent dementia:

1. Never stop learning. Stimulate your mind. The rewards are boundless. Learning new things will excite you and open up possibilities you never knew existed. An appetite for knowledge will keep your brain young.

2. Keep your blood vessels healthy so they can deliver oxygen and nutrients to your brain efficiently and remove cellular waste.

3. Stimulate all of your senses: sight, sound, touch, taste, and smell. Look at the beauty around you: nature, people, art, and music. We are surrounded by beauty. It's time to take notice. God created us and the world around us. These creations are beautiful. Take notice and enjoy them and be forever grateful for this gift.

4. Listen to the beauty around you. The sounds of people, nature, and music. What a joy! Imagine what it would be like without this.

5. Reach out and touch someone. It feels good. Touch is one of the oldest forms of communication.

6. Relish the taste of natural, wholesome foods including fruits, vegetables, and nuts. They contain the antioxidants and phytonutrients needed for optimal health.

7. Take in the smells of nature: flowers, forests, plants, oceans, and the wonderful smells after a rain.

8. We live in a beautiful world. Take in the gifts it is giving you, and you will rejuvenate in mind, body, spirit, and soul.

9. Live a life of gratitude; it will bring you happiness. In my experience, happy people live longer with less cognitive decline.

10. Reduce chronic inflammation. Cognitive decline is directly related to chronic inflammation of not just the brain but the body as a whole. This is a major player in dementia and chronic diseases in general. Control inflammation, and you may live forever, including your brain.

11. Maintaining youthful hormonal balance is critical to good health, especially the health of your brain.

12. Keeping the body moving with exercise keeps the brain moving.

13. Don't smoke; this is an obvious one. If you are reading this book, then chances are you are not a smoker. Smoking is a sure way to get dementia and die. There are few things worse for your health than smoking. There is absolutely nothing good about smoking. It is all negative.

14. Control your blood pressure; be sure to have your doctor check your blood pressure on a regular basis. It is easy to treat in most cases. High blood pressure will cause damage to your blood vessels, reducing blood flow to your brain, heart, and all organs of your body.

15. Get hearing aids as soon as possible if your hearing is impaired. Your brain needs all of the stimulation it can get, especially sound.

16. Control your weight. It will reduce inflammation, and you will be healthier for it. Remember, belly fat is especially inflammatory, so work on getting rid of that roll.

17. Develop and enjoy a great social life. Life is more fun when you share it with others, and your brain will love you for it.

18. Don't get diabetes. Diabetes will cause accelerated aging and increase your chances of getting dementia. Adopting healthy lifestyle habits will minimize this risk.

REFERENCES
FOR NUTRITION
CHAPTER

Agren JJ, Hanninen O, Julkunen A, et al. Fish diet, fish oil and do-cosahexaenoic acid rich oil lower fasting and postprandial plasma lipid levels. Eur J Clin Nutr 1996;50:765–71.

Alpaslan M, Gunduz H. The effects of growing conditions on oil content, fatty acid composition and tocopherol content of some sunflower varieties produced in Turkey. Die Nahrung (Germany) 2000; 44(6):434–7.

Am J Clin Nutr. 2004;79(3):362–71.

Am J Clin Nutr. 2004;79(3):362–71.

Armas LA, Hollis BW, Heaney RP. Vitamin D2 is much less effective than vitamin D3 in humans. J Clin Endocrinol Metab. 2004;89(11):5387–91.

Arunabh S, Pollack S, Yeh J, Aloia JF. Body fat content and 25-hydroxyvitamin D levels in healthy women. J Clin Endocrinol Metab. 2003;88(1):157–61.

Barta DJ, Tibbitts TW, Barta DJ. Calcium localization and tip-burn development in lettuce leaves during early enlargement. Journal of the American Society for Horticultural Science 2000; 125(3):294–8.

Bertone-Johnson ER, Hankinson SE, Bendich A, et al. Calcium and vitamin D intake and risk of incident premenstrual syndrome. Arch Intern Med 2005;165:1246–52.

Bischoff HA, Stahelin HB, Dick W, et al. Effects of vitamin D and calcium supplementation on falls: a randomized controlled trial. J Bone Miner Res 2003;18:343–51.

Bischoff-Ferrari HA, Dawson-Hughes B, Willett WC, et al. Effect of Vitamin D on falls: a meta-analysis. JAMA 2004;291:1999–2006.

Bischoff-Ferrari HA, Giovannucci E, Willett WC, Dietrich T, Dawson-Hughes B. Estimation of optimal serum concentrations of 25-hydroxyvitamin D for multiple health outcomes. Am J Clin Nutr. 2006;84(1):18–28.

Bischoff-Ferrari HA, Willett WC, Wong JB, Giovannucci E, Dietrich T, Dawson-Hughes B. Fracture prevention with vitamin D supplementation: a meta-analysis of randomized controlled trials. JAMA. 2005;293(18):2257–64.

Blumberg J. Public health implications of preventive nutrition. In: Bendich A, Deckelbaum RJ, Editors. Preventive Nutrition. Humana Press, Totowa, NJ, 1997.

Borissova AM, Tankova T, Kirilov G, Dakovska L, Kovacheva R. The effect of vitamin D3 on insulin secretion and peripheral insulin sensitivity in type 2 diabetic patients. Int J Clin Pract. 2003;57(4):258–61.

Bottino NR. Lipid composition of two species of Antarctic krill: Euphausia superba and E. crystallorophias. Comp Biochem Physiol B 1975;50:479–84.

Bowman BB, Rosenberg IH. Assessment of the Nutritional Status of the Elderly. American Journal of Clinical Nutrition 1982; 35(5 Suppl):1142–51.

Burdge GC, Jones AE, Wootton SA. Eicosapentaenoic and docosapentaenoic acids are the principal products of alpha-linolenic acid metabolism in young men. Br J Nutr. 2002;88(4):355–64.

Burdge GC, Wootton SA. Conversion of alpha-linolenic acid to eicosapentaenoic, docosapentaenoic and docosahexaenoic acids in young women. Br J Nutr. 2002;88(4):411–20.

Calder PC. n-3 polyunsaturated fatty acids, inflammation, and inflammatory diseases. Am J Clin Nutr. 2006;83:1505S–1519S.

Calton JB. Prevalence of Micronutrient Deficiency in Popular Diet Plans. JISSN. 2010;7:24

Chapuy MC, Preziosi P, Maamer M, et al. Prevalence of vitamin D insufficiency in an adult normal population. Osteoporos Int. 1997;7(5):439–43.

Cho E, Hung S, Willet W, et al. Prospective study of dietary fat and the risk of age-related macular degeneration. Am J Clin Nutr. 2001;73:209–18.

Church TS, Earnest CP, Wood KA. James B. Kampert. Reduction of C-Reactive Protein Levels Throughthrough Use of a Multivitamin. Am J Med. 2003;115:702–7.

Composition of Foods: Raw, Processed, Prepared. USDA National Nutrient Database for Standard Reference, Release 15. December 2002. U.S.US Department of Agriculture, Agricultural Research Service, Beltsville Human Nutrition Research Center, Nutrient Data Laboratory.

CRN Reacts to Institute of Medicine DRI Recommendations for Vitamin D. November 30, 2010. Retrieved December 6, 2010 from https://www.crnusa.org/CRNPR10_CRNVitDDRIresp113010.html.

Culp TM. Vitamins and HIV Therapy: A Naturopathic Perspective. STEP perspective 1995; 7(1):1,7.

Danaei G, Ding EL, Mozaffarian D, et al. The Preventable Causes of Death in the United States: Comparative Risk Assessment of Dietary, Lifestyle, and Metabolic Risk Factors. PLoS Med. 2009 Apr 28;6(4):e1000058.

Datz T. Harvard Serves Up Its Own "'Plate.'" Harvard Gazette. September 14, 2011. Retrieved April 30, 2014 from http://news.harvard.edu/gazette/story/2011/09/harvard-serves-up-its-own-plate/?utm_content.

Davis B. Essential Fatty Acids in Vegetarian Nutrition. Andrews University Nutrition Department. Accessed August 18, 2005 from http://www.andrews.edu/NUFS/essentialfat.htm.

den Heijer M, Brouwer IA, Bos GM, et al. Vitamin supplementation reduces blood homocysteine levels: a controlled trial in patients with venous thrombosis and healthy volunteers. Arterioscler Thromb Vasc Biol. 1998 Mar;18(3):356–61.

Diet quality of Americans in 2001–02 and 2007–08 as measured by the Healthy Eating Index-2010. Nutrition Insight 51. USDA Center for Nutrition Policy and Promotion. April 2013.

Dunlap WC, Fujisawa A, Yamamoto Y, et al. Notothenioid fish, krill and phytoplankton from Antarctica contain a vitamin E constituent (alpha-tocomonoenol) functionally associated with cold-water adaptation. Comp Biochem Physiol B Biochem Mol Biol 2002;133:299–305.

Earnest CP, Wood KA, Church TS. Complex multivitamin supplementation improves homocysteine and resistance to LDL-C oxidation. J Am Coll Nutr. 2003;22(5):400–407.

Feskanich D, Willett WC, Colditz GA. Calcium, vitamin D, milk consumption, and hip fractures: a prospective study among postmenopausal women. Am J Clin Nutr. 2003;77(2):504–11.

Fletcher RH, Fairfield KM. Vitamins for chronic disease prevention in adults. JAMA 2002; 287(23):3127–9.

Food and Nutrition Board, Institute of Medicine. Vitamin D. Dietary Reference Intakes: Calcium, Phosphorus, Magnesium, Vitamin D, and Fluoride. Washington D.C.: National Academies Press; 1999:250–87.

Forrest KY, Stuhldreher WL. Prevalence and correlates of vitamin D deficiency in US adults. Nutr Res. 2011;31(1):48–54.

Fortin PR, Lew RA, Liang MH, et al. Validation of a meta-analysis: the effects of fish oil in rheumatoid arthritis. J Clin Epidemiol. 1995;48(11):1379–90.

Gaziano JM, Sesso HD, Christen WG, Bubes V, Smith JP, MacFadyen J, Schvartz M, Manson JE, Glynn RJ, Buring JE. Multivitamins in the prevention of cancer in men: the Physicians' Health Study II randomized controlled trial. JAMA. 2012 Nov 14;308(18):1871-80.

Gerrior, S. and Bente, L. 1997. Nutrient content of the US Food Supply, 1909–94. US Department of Agriculture, Center for Nutrition Policy and Promotion. Home Economics Report No. 53.

Ginde AA, Liu MC, Camargo CA Jr. Demographic differences and trends of vitamin D insufficiency in the US population, 1988–2004. Arch Intern Med. 2009;169:626–32.

Gorham ED, Garland CF, Garland FC, et al. Vitamin D and prevention of colorectal cancer. J Steroid Biochem Mol Biol. 2005;97(1–2):179–94.

Griffin MD, Xing N, Kumar R. Vitamin D and its analogs as regulators of immune activation and antigen presentation. Annu Rev Nutr. 2003;23:117–45.

Hamazaki T, Hirayama S. The effect of docosahexaenoic acid-containing food administration on symptoms of attention-deficit/hyperactivity disorder-a placebo-controlled double-blind study. Eur J Clin Nutr. 2004;58:838.

Harris SS, Soteriades E, Coolidge JA, Mudgal S, Dawson-Hughes B. Vitamin D insufficiency and hyperparathyroidism in a low income, multiracial, elderly population. J Clin Endocrinol Metab. 2000;85(11):4125–30.

Harris WS. n-3 fatty acids and serum lipoproteins: human studies. Am J Clin Nutr. 1997;65(5 Suppl):1645S–1654S.

Hayes CE, Nashold FE, Spach KM, Pedersen LB. The immunological functions of the vitamin D endocrine system. Cell Mol Biol. 2003;49(2):277–300.

Heaney RP, Dowell MS, Hale CA, Bendich A. Calcium absorption varies within the reference range for serum 25-hydroxyvitamin D. J Am Coll Nutr. 2003;22(2):142–6.

Heaney RP. Long-latency deficiency disease: insights from calcium and vitamin D. Am J Clin Nutr. 2003;78(5):912–19.

Higdon J, Drake VJ, DeLuca HF. Vitamin D. The Linus Pauling Institute Micronutrient Information Center 2000- 2010; Last updated 11/30/10. Retrieved December 6, 2010 from http://lpi.oregonstate.edu/infocenter/vitamins/vitaminD/.

Holick MF. Vitamin D deficiency. N Engl J Med. 2007;357(3):266–81.

Holick MF. Vitamin D deficiency: what a pain it is. Mayo Clin Proc. 2003;78(12):1457–9.

Holick MF. Vitamin D: A millenium perspective. J Cell Biochem. 2003;88(2):296–307.

Holick MF. Vitamin D: importance in the prevention of cancers, type 1 diabetes, heart disease, and osteoporosis. Am J Clin Nutr. 2004;79(3):362–71.

Holmquist C, Larsson S, Wolk A, de Faire U. Multivitamin Supplements Are Inversely Associated with Risk of Myocardial Infarction in Men and Women—Stockholm Heart. Epidemiology Program (SHEEP). J Nutr. 2003;133: 2650–4.

Hoogendijk WJG, Lips P, Dik MG, Deeg DJH, Beekman ATF, Penninx BWJH. Depression is associated with decreased 25-hydroxyvitamin D and increased parathyroid hormone levels in older adults. Archives of General Psychiatry 2008; 65(5):495.

Hou TZ, Mooneyham RE. Applied studies of plant meridian system: I. The effect of agri-wave technology on yield and quality of tomato. American Journal of Chinese medicine 1999; 27(1):1–10.

Hu FB, Bronner L, Willett WC, et al. Fish and omega-3 fatty acid intake and risk of coronary heart disease in women. JAMA. 2002;287(14):1815–21.

Huskisson E, Maggini S, Ruf M. The role of vitamins and minerals in energy metabolism and well-being. J Int Med Res. 2007 May–Jun;35(3):277–89.

Inomata S, Kadowaki S, Yamatani T, Fukase M, Fujita T. Effect of 1 alpha (OH)-vitamin D3 on insulin secretion in diabetes mellitus. Bone Miner. 1986;1(3):187–92.

Jahnsen J, Falch JA, Mowinckel P, Aadland E. Vitamin D status, parathyroid hormone and bone mineral density in patients with inflammatory bowel disease. Scand J Gastroenterol. 2002;37(2):192–9.

Jarvinen R, Knekt P, Rissanen H, Reunanen A. Intake of fish and long-chain n-3 fatty acids and the risk of coronary heart mortality in men and women. Br J Nutr. 2006;95(4):824–9.

Jones PJH, Papamandjaris AA. "Chapter 10—Lipids: Cellular Metabolism" In: Present Knowledge in Nutrition, 8th ed. Bowman BA, Russell RM (eds). Washington, DC: ILSI Press; 2001:104–14.

Kris-Etherton PM, Harris WS, Appel LJ. Fish consumption, fish oil, omega-3 fatty acids, and cardiovascular disease. Circulation. 2002;106(21):2747–57.

Kubota J, Allaway WH. Geographic distribution of trace element problems. In J.J. Mortvedt, ed., Micronutrients in Agriculture: Proceedings of Symposium held at Muscle Shoals, Alabama, Madison, WI: Soil Science Society of America; 1972:525–54.

Li YC, Kong J, Wei M, Chen ZF, Liu SQ, Cao LP. 1,25-Dihydroxyvitamin D(3) is a negative endocrine regulator of the renin-angiotensin system. J Clin Invest. 2002;110(2):229–38.

Lieberman S, Bruning N. The Real Vitamin & Mineral Book, Second Edition. Garden City Park, New York: Avery Publishing Group; 1997:26.

Lin R, White JH. The pleiotropic actions of vitamin D. Bioessays. 2004;26(1):21–8.

Long SJ, Benton D. Effects of vitamin and mineral supplementation on stress, mild psychiatric symptoms, and mood in nonclinical samples: a meta-analysis. Psychosom Med. 2013 Feb;75(2):144–53.

Lovaza: Omega-3 Acid Ethyl Esters. Retrieved August 6, 2009 from http://www.lovaza.com/index.html?banner_s=208381923&rotation_s=30492788.

Lucas M, Asselin G, Merette C, et al. Effects of ethyl-eicosapentaenoic acid omega-3 fatty acid supplementation on hot flashes and quality of life among middle-aged women: a double-blind, placebo-controlled, randomized clinical trial. Menopause. 2009;16:357–66.

Malabanan A, Veronikis IE, Holick MF. Redefining vitamin D insufficiency. Lancet. 1998;351(9105):805–6.

McGinnis JM, Ernst ND. Preventive nutrition: A historic perspective and future economic outlook. In: Bendich A, Deckelbaum RJ, Editors. Primary and Secondary Preventive Nutrition. Humana Press, Totowa, NJ, 2001.

McKeehen JD, Smart DJ, Mackowiak CL, et al. Effect of CO_2 levels on nutrient content of lettuce and radish. Advances in space research: the official journal of the Committee on Space Research 1996; 18(4–5):85–92.

MedlinePlus. Fish Oil. U.S.US National Library of Medicine. Last reviewed—12/10/2011. Retrieved August 29, 2012 from http://www.nlm.nih.gov/medlineplus/druginfo/natural/993.html.

Merlino LA, Curtis J, Mikuls TR, et al. Vitamin D intake is inversely associated with rheumatoid arthritis. Arthritis Rheum 2004;50:72–7.

Mori TA, Burke V, Puddey IB, et al. Purified eicosapentaenoic and docosahexaenoic acids have differential effects on serum lipids and lipoproteins, LDL particle size, glucose, and insulin in mildly hyperlipidemic men. Am J Clin Nutr 2000;71:1085–94.

Morris MC, Evans DA, Bienias JL, et al. Consumption of fish and n-3 fatty acids and risk of incident Alzheimer disease. Arch Neurol. 2003;60:940–6.

Munger KL, Zhang SM, O'Reilly E, et al. Vitamin D intake and incidence of multiple sclerosis. Neurology 2004;62:60–5.

Murphy SP, White KK, Park SY, Sharma S. Multivitamin-multimineral supplements' effect on total nutrient intake. Am J Clin Nutr. 2007 Jan;85(1):280S–284S.

Murray MT. Encyclopedia of Nutritional Supplements. Rocklin, CA: Prima Health; 1996:9.

Nesby-O'Dell S, Scanlon KS, Cogswell ME, et al. Hypovitaminosis D prevalence and determinants among African American and white women of reproductive age: third National Health and Nutrition Examination Survey, 1988–1994. Am J Clin Nutr. 2002;76(1):187–92.

Prisco D, Paniccia R, Bandinelli B, et al. Effect of medium-term supplementation with a moderate dose of n-3 polyunsaturated fatty acids on blood pressure in mild hypertensive patients. Thromb Res 1998;1:105–12.

Rautiainen S, Akesson A, Levitan EB, Morgenstern R, Mittleman MA, Wolk A. Multivitamin Use and the Risk of Myocardial Infarction: A Population-Based Cohort of Swedish Women. Am J Clin Nutr. 2010 Nov;92(5):1251–6.

Report Card on the Quality of Americans' Diets. Nutrition insights, INSIGHT 28. USDA Center for Nutrition Policy and Promotion. December 2002.

Simopoulos AP. The importance of the ratio of omega-6/omega-3 essential fatty acids. Biomed Pharmacother. 2002;56(8):365–79.

Stevens LJ, Zentall SS, Deck JL, et al. Essential fatty acid metabolism in boys with attention-deficit hyperactivity disorder. Am J Clin Nutr. 1995;62:761–8.

Suarez EC. Plasma interleukin-6 is associated with psychological coronary risk factors: moderation by use of multivitamin supplements. Brain Behav Immun. 2003 Aug;17(4):296–303.

Sweet L. Michelle Obama Hypes Icon Switch: Bye food pyramid, Hello Food Plate. Transcript. June 2, 2011. Chicago Sun-Times. Retrieved April 30, 2014.

Tangpricha V, Koutkia P, Rieke SM, Chen TC, Perez AA, Holick MF. Fortification of orange juice with vitamin D: a novel approach for enhancing vitamin D nutritional health. Am J Clin Nutr. 2003;77(6):1478–83.

The Centers for Disease Control and Prevention's Division of Laboratory Sciences at the National Center for Environmental Health. Second National Report on Biochemical Indicators of Diet and Nutrition in the U.S.US Population 2012. Executive Summary. Retrieved August 19, 2014 from http://www.cdc.gov/nutritionreport/pdf/exesummary_web_032612.pdf.

Thomas MK, Lloyd-Jones DM, Thadhani RI, et al. Hypovitaminosis D in medical inpatients. N Engl J Med. 1998;338(12):777–83.

Thurnham D. Red cell enzyme tests of vitamin status: Do marginal deficiencies have any physiological significance? Proceedings of the Nutrition Society 1981; 40(2):155–63.

Toft I, Bonaa KH, Ingebretsen OC, et al. Effects of n-3 polyunsaturated fatty acids on glucose homeostasis and blood pressure in essential hypertension. A randomized, controlled trial. Ann Intern Med 1995;123:911–18.

Ulven SM, Kirkhus B, Lamglait A, Basu S, Elind E, Haider T, Berge K, Vik H, Pedersen JI. Metabolic effects of krill oil are essentially similar to those of fish oil but at lower dose of EPA and DHA, in healthy volunteers. Lipids 2011;46(1):37–46.

Understanding Vitamin D Cholecalciferol. The Vitamin D Council, n.d., Retrieved December 6, 2010 from http://www.vitamindcouncil.org/.

United States Department of Agriculture, Center for Nutrition Policy and Promotion. MyPlate. Last Modified: 12/11/2013. Retrieved April 30, 2014 from http://www.cnpp.usda.gov/myplate.htm.

United States Department of Agriculture. Center for Nutrition Policy and Promotion/ Comparison of Nutrient Content of each Each 2010 USDA Food Pattern to Nutritional Goals for that Pattern. Retrieved August 19, 2014 from http://www.cnpp.usda.gov/Publications/USDAFoodPatterns/ComparisonofNutrientContentofeach2010USDAFood PatterntoNutritionalGoalsforthatPattern.pdf.

USDA National Nutrient Database for Standard Reference, Release 15 , USDA Nutrient Data Laboratory, Last updated December 11, 2002; http://www.nal.usda.gov/fnic/foodcomp/.

Vaughan CP, Johnson TM 2nd, Goode PS, Redden DT, Burgio KL, Markland AD. Vitamin D and lower urinary tract symptoms among US men: results from the 2005–2006 National Health and Nutrition Examination Survey. Urology. 2011 Dec;78(6):1292–7.

Vereshagin AG and Novitskaya GV. The triglyceride composition of linseed oil. Journal of the American Oil Chemists' Society 1965;42:970–4.

Vieth R. Vitamin D supplementation, 25-hydroxyvitamin D concentrations, and safety. Am J Clin Nutr. 1999;69(5):842–56.

Voigt RG, Llorente AM, Jensen CL, et al. A randomized, double-blind, placebo-controlled trial of docosahexaenoic acid supplementation in children with attention-deficit/hyperactivity disorder. J Pediatr. 2001;139:189–96.

Wagner CL, Greer FR, and the Section on Breastfeeding and Committee on Nutrition. Prevention of rickets and vitamin D deficiency in infants, children, and adolescents. American Academy of Pediatrics. 2008;122(5):1142–52.

Wall R, Ross RP, Fitzgerald GF, Stanton C. Fatty acids from fish: the anti-inflammatory potential of long-chain omega-3 fatty acids. Nutr Rev. 2010;68(5):280–9.

Wang C, Harris WS, Chung M, et al. n-3 Fatty acids from fish or fish-oil supplements, but not alpha-linolenic acid, benefit cardiovascular disease outcomes in primary- and secondary-prevention studies: a systematic review. Am J Clin Nutr. 2006;84(1):5–17.

Wang C, Li Y, Zhu K, Dong YM, Sun CH. Effects of Supplementation with Multivitamin and Mineral on Blood Pressure and C-reactive Protein in Obese Chinese Women with Increased Cardiovascular Disease Risk. Asia Pac J Clin Nutr. 2009;18(1):121–30.

Ward E. Addressing nutritional gaps with multivitamin and mineral supplements. Nutr J. 2014 Jul 15;13(1):72.

Wharton B, Bishop N. Rickets. Lancet. 2003;362(9393):1389–1400.

Whitney EN, Cataldo CB, Rolfes SR. Understanding Normal and Clinical Nutrition, 5th ed. Belmont, CA:West/Wadsworth; 1998:141–175.

Xu Q, Parks CG, DeRoo LA, Cawthon RM, Sandler DP, Chen H. Multivitamin use and telomere length in women. Am J Clin Nutr. 2009;89(6):1857–63.

Yosefy C, Viskoper JR, Laszt A, et al. The effect of fish oil on hypertension, plasma lipids and hemostasis in hypertensive, obese, dyslipidemic patients with and without diabetes mellitus. Prostaglandins Leukot Essent Fatty Acids 1999;61:83–7.

Zeitz U, Weber K, Soegiarto DW, Wolf E, Balling R, Erben RG. Impaired insulin secretory capacity in mice lacking a functional vitamin D receptor. FASEB J. 2003;17(3):509–11.

Zittermann A. Vitamin D in preventive medicine: are we ignoring the evidence? Br J Nutr. 2003;89(5):552–72.

REFERENCES
FOR EXERCISE
CHAPTER

ACSM's Guidelines for Exercise Testing and Prescription. Philadelphia: Wolters Kluwer/Lippincott Williams & Wilkins Health, 2014. Print.

Baechle, Thomas R., and Roger W. Earle. Essentials of Strength Training and Conditioning. 3rd ed. Champaign, IL: Human Kinetics, 2008. Print.

Bushman, Barbara A. "Exercise and Sleep." ACSM's Health & Fitness Journal 17.5 (2013): 5–8. Web.

Craft, Lynette L., and Frank M. Perna. "The Benefits of Exercise for the Clinically Depressed." The Primary Care Companion to The Journal of Clinical Psychiatry 06.03 (2004): 104–11. Web.

Garber, Carol Ewing, Bryan Blissmer, Michael R. Deschenes, Barry A. Franklin, Michael J. Lamonte, I-Min Lee, David C. Nieman, and David P. Swain. "Quantity and Quality of Exercise for Developing and Maintaining Cardiorespiratory, Musculoskeletal, and for Neuromotor Fitness in Apparently Healthy Adults." Medicine & Science in Sports & Exercise 43.7 (2011): 1334–59. Web. 4 May 2017.

Iftikhar, Imran H., Christopher E. Kline, and Shawn D. Youngst-edt. "Effects of Exercise Training on Sleep Apnea: A Meta-analysis." Lung 192.1 (2013): 175–84. Web.

"Prevalence of Self-Reported Obesity among US Adults by State and Territory, BRFSS, 2015." Centers for Disease Control and Prevention. N.p., n.d. Web. 18 May 2017.

ABOUT THE
AUTHOR

Dr. Jacob Rosenstein is an author and speaker, who is passionate about helping people get well. He is a board-certified neurosurgeon and diplomate of the American Board of Neurological Surgery as well as a Fellow of the American College of Surgeons. Dr. Rosenstein is the founder of North Texas Neurosurgical Consultants and Southwest Age Intervention Institute in the Dallas/ Fort Worth Metroplex. He has been in private practice since 1985 and specializes in neurological surgery and age management/ anti-aging medicine. Famous for his amazing transformation in aging in his own life, he has been featured in various media, TV shows, advertisements, and articles for his commitment to taking control of his health. He wrote and starred in The Dr. R Show, a TV series on health and wellness.

Dr. Rosenstein has an illustrious career and credentials including:

BA degree in human biology from Johns Hopkins University where he was Phi Beta Kappa.

Medical degree from The Johns Hopkins University School of Medicine where he was Alpha Omega Alpha.

Residency in Neurological Surgery at UT Southwestern Medical Center/Parkland Hospital in Dallas.

Chief resident of Neurological Surgery at UT Southwestern Medical Center/Parkland Hospital in Dallas.

Fellowship training in Neurosurgery at the Institute of Neurology, Department of Neurosurgery, at the National Hospital for Nervous Diseases in London, England

Cenegenics Education & Research Foundation Age Management Medicine Training and Certification.

Notes

Notes

Notes

Notes

Notes

Notes

HOW IS THIS NEUROSURGEON YOUNGER THAN HIS OWN SON?

Meet Dr. Jacob Rosenstein, world-renowned neurosurgeon and inventor of Vitamere™. His calendar age is 62, but his biologic age is less than 20. This is measured by his mean telomere length.

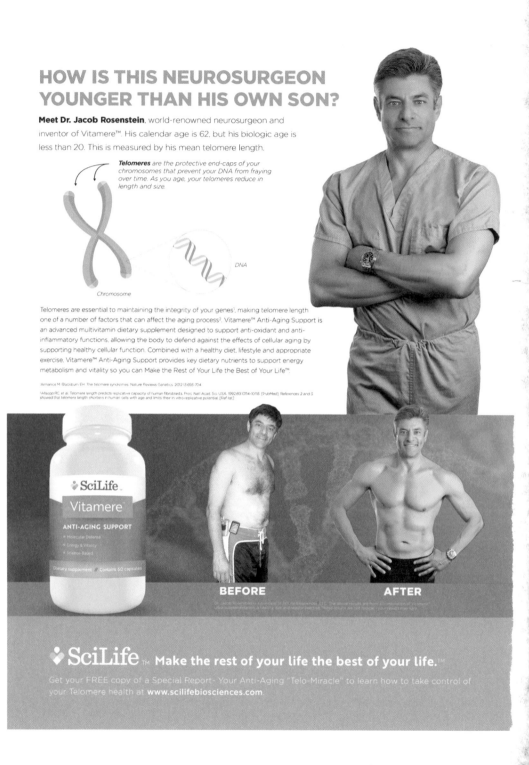

Telomeres are the protective end-caps of your chromosomes that prevent your DNA from fraying over time. As you age, your telomeres reduce in length and size.

DNA

Chromosome

Telomeres are essential to maintaining the integrity of your genes[1], making telomere length one of a number of factors that can affect the aging process[2]. Vitamere™ Anti-Aging Support is an advanced multivitamin dietary supplement designed to support anti-oxidant and anti-inflammatory functions, allowing the body to defend against the effects of cellular aging by supporting healthy cellular function. Combined with a healthy diet, lifestyle and appropriate exercise, Vitamere™ Anti-Aging Support provides key dietary nutrients to support energy metabolism and vitality so you can Make the Rest of Your Life the Best of Your Life™.

Armanios M, Blackburn EH. The telomere syndromes. Nature Reviews Genetics. 2012 13:693-704

[1]Allsopp RC et al. Telomere length predicts replicative capacity of human fibroblasts. Proc Natl Acad Sci USA. 1992;89:10114-10118. [PubMed] References 2 and 3 showed that telomere length shortens in human cells with age and limits their in vitro replicative potential. [Ref list]

SciLife
Vitamere
ANTI-AGING SUPPORT
- Molecular Defense
- Energy & Vitality
- Science Based

Dietary supplement / Contains 60 capsules

BEFORE

AFTER

Dr. Jacob Rosenstein is a product of his lifestyle. The above results are from a combination of Vitamere™ ultra supplementation, a healthy diet and regular exercise. These results are not typical - your results may vary.

◆ SciLife ™ Make the rest of your life the best of your life.™

Get your FREE copy of a Special Report- Your Anti-Aging "Telo-Miracle" to learn how to take control of your Telomere health at **www.scilifebiosciences.com**.